Without Child

WITHOUT CHILD
Experiencing and Resolving Infertility

by
Ellen Sarasohn Glazer

and

Susan Lewis Cooper

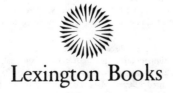

Lexington Books

D.C. Heath and Company · Lexington, Massachusetts · Toronto

"Rosegardens and Fertile Valleys," by Sally Chapralis is reprinted with permission of RESOLVE of Chicago newsletter, January 1986.

"I Met a Woman Yesterday" is excerpted with permission from Katherine Schneider Aker and *Mothering* Magazine, Mother Poet, published by John McMahon and Peggy O'Mara McMahon, PO Box 1690, Santa Fe, NM 87504. All rights reserved.

"Can Anyone Understand?" is reprinted with permission from the author. © Louise Fulton, 1988.

Thank you to *Lilith*, the Jewish women's magazine, 250 W. 57th Street #2432, New York, NY 10107, for permission to reprint "Infertile, Male, and Jewish."

"Prayerem," is reprinted with permission from the author. © Jean DeMers Gilroy. 1987.

"Stillbirth" is excerpted with permission from Barbara Crooker and *Mothering* Magazine, Mother Poet, published by John McMahon and Peggy O'Mara McMahon, PO Box 1690, Santa Fe, NM 87504. All rights reserved.

"Taps in the Cabbage Patch" is reprinted with permission from the author. © Terri Flynn, 1987.

"The Mother of My Child" was originally published in *13th Moon* and in *Motherwriter*, poems by Judith Steinbergh (Wampeter, 1983). Reprinted with permission.

"The Adoption," is reprinted with permission. © Fran Castan.

The authors gratefully acknowledge Perspectives Press for permitting the reprint of "Mother's Day," previously published in *Perspective on a Grafted Tree*, by Margaret Munk.

Library of Congress Cataloging-in-Publication Data

Without child

1. Infertility – Popular works. 2. Infertility –
Psychological aspects. I. Glazer, Ellen. II. Cooper,
Susan, 1947 –
RC889.W575   1988   616.6'92   87 – 45732
ISBN 0 – 669 – 16889 – 0 (alk. paper).
ISBN 0 – 669 – 21363 – 2 (pbk. : alk. paper)

Published simultaneously in Canada
Printed in the United States of America
Casebound International Standard Book Number: 0 – 669 – 16889 – 0
Paperbound International Standard Book Number: 0 – 669 – 21362 – 2
Library of Congress Catalog Card Number: 87 – 45732

The paper used in this publication meets
the minimum requirements of American National Standard
for Information Sciences – Permanence of Paper
for Printed Library Materials, ANSI Z39.48 – 1984.

89 90 91 92 8 7 6 5 4 3

Contents

This book is dedicated to our parents,
Ira Sarasohn and Shirlee Sarasohn and
Doris and Allen Lewis, who conceived us,
guided us, and delight in our accomplishments;
and to Elizabeth and Mollie Glazer and
Seth and Amanda Cooper, our long awaited
children, who are the seeds from which this book
has grown.

Preface and Acknowledgments

I T is with pride and a sense of accomplishment that we complete the task of writing this book. It has had a long gestation. Although we did not know it at the time, it was conceived nearly ten years ago, shortly after we met through RESOLVE, Inc. Ellen had come to Susan's office to get a copy of her doctoral dissertation about the emotional impact of infertility. The two of us began talking about Susan's research, then launched into personal accounts of our own infertility. The sharing that occurred then, and that we have seen time and again in our work as RESOLVE Support group leaders, forms the foundation for this book.

We are now working mothers. Susan has two biological children, ages eleven and seven. She was treated for both primary and secondary infertility. Ellen has two children, one adopted and one biological, ages seven and four. We have both experienced pregnancy losses. Our lives, to varying degrees, are filled with many child-oriented activities. Raising children is more difficult than we thought, yet we are grateful for the privilege of mother-hood. Still, we remember the loneliness, the pain, and the longings we felt when we were so desperately trying to conceive. We remember that it helped to read about infertility, though there was little available, and to talk with others who understood. We wrote this book in order to provide comfort, support, and guidance to all who suffer from the ache of infertility and to educate those who are unaware of this suffering.

The process of writing and editing this book has been immensely satisfying. It has given us an opportunity to pull together much of what we have learned from our clients, from friends, and from our own experience. It has prompted us to keep up with the rapid medical and technological advances in the field of reproductive medicine. It has also given us a greater appreciation of the ways in which people can emerge from a crisis whole—having suffered, and having grown. And finally, it has given us a wonderful opportunity to become closer friends—to continue developing a relationship that was conceived from the pain of our infertility and nourished by a joint creative endeavor.

We are keenly aware as we complete this book, that it would never have come to fruition without the help and resources of so many people. We deeply appreciate their efforts. Our fifty contributors—poets and authors—are the people to whom we are especially indebted. It is obvious that without their work, a book of this nature could never have been written. Their varied experiences and perspectives offer a richness and dimension that we have not previously discovered in a book about infertility. We thank them deeply.

Though she probably knows nothing of this endeavor, we must begin by thanking Barbara Eck Menning, founder of RESOLVE, Inc. Her foresight and perseverance led to the formation of a large national organization that offers support, medical information, and advocacy to infertile people. Without RESOLVE, Susan could never have written her specific doctoral dissertation, and the two of us most likely would not have met. Without RESOLVE, we probably would not have become support group leaders, nor developed skills in working with infertile patients. Thus we could never have written this book. And, without RESOLVE, we would not have had access to all the people who so willingly sent us essays and poetry.

Perhaps most important, we wish to thank the hundreds of infertile men and women who have crossed our paths in the last ten years—friends, colleagues, support group members, and patients. Though we have certainly drawn on our own experience in writing this book, it is they who have been our invaluable teachers. We hope that this book reflects their experiences, wisdom, pain, good humor, and courage. They have surely enriched us, both personally and professionally.

Numerous other people helped in various ways and we would like to acknowledge them, though in no particular order of importance. Beverly Freeman offered us the resources of the RESOLVE office and, in the final stages of the book, provided us with much useful marketing advice. Joan Jack also offered us encouragement, practical advice, and marketing help when we needed it. Authors Linda Salzer and Carol Kort gave us initial advice, support, and encouragement about publication. Judith Steinbergh—poet, author, songwriter—first introduced us to many of the poems that appear in this book.

We would like to thank Don Glazer for suggesting we write this book. We thank Judy Chiel for putting us in touch with Lexington Books. And we would like to give special thanks to Margaret Zusky, our editor, who has been a continual source of encouragement to us. Her enthusiasm about the material we regularly sent her spurred us on to collect and produce more.

Two people provided medical expertise when we needed it: Diane Clapp was always available to answer the many questions we had, prior to our writing the more technical chapters, and Gary Gross readily agreed to be our "medical editor" when the manuscript was completed. We thank them both for their help.

Four people took care of our manuscript. Louise MacDonald and Winnie Carroll did much of the typing. We thank them for their careful work. Ivy Feuerstadt and Nelson Wasserman deserve special thanks for housing an extra copy of the manuscript, just in case both our houses burned down on the same day. Fortunately, we did not need the extra copy, but knowing it was there made us feel more secure.

Ellen would like to thank Ellen Kleiner of *Mothering Magazine*, Santa Fe, New Mexico, a lifelong friend who graciously offered the resources of her magazine. She thanks, too, Danny Gottsegen, a longtime friend, whose support and encouragement were greatly appreciated when this project was in its early stages. Ellen would also like to say thank you to her children, Elizabeth and Mollie, for their understanding and cooperation, particularly when she broke her leg in the home stretch of this endeavor. And finally she would like to thank Ann Woodfork who, for her, will always be the stork.

Susan thanks her husband, Marc, for convincing her that her "computer phobia" was all in her head, and that she could indeed learn how to use a word processor. She thanks Marc, as well as her children, Seth and Amanda, for (only sometimes reluctantly) leaving the computer site when they saw her approach. And finally, she thanks John Shane, her former infertility specialist, who moved to Oklahoma a few months after she conceived. Although she has not seen him in almost twelve years, and he has undoubtedly forgotten her, his kindness, empathy, and respect for his patients have remained with her as a model for the doctor-patient relationship.

I met a woman yesterday,
she had a tiny baby, the
baby had been born without one
hand. I wondered if she had
thanked God for her baby.

Katherine Schneider Aker

Introduction:
Infertility, A Dawning Realization

Susie and Jimmy sitting in a tree,
K-I-S-S-I-N-G
First comes love, then comes marriage,
Then comes the baby in the baby carriage.

THIS familiar childhood jingle reinforces the notion that babies are the natural result of love and marriage. Thus, it is not surprising that most couples assume that parenthood will come easily—the natural outcome of their loving relationship. They approach conception with delight and with optimism. The child they create will symbolize their joy; it will be their legacy.

The birth control pill, and to a somewhat lesser extent the IUD, heralded the age of dependable planned parenthood. And with it, the element of timing was added to the love-plus-marriage-equals-baby equation. Most couples today, unlike their parents and grandparents, do not worry about conceiving a child before they are emotionally and financially able to do so.

When a couple finally does decide to become parents, they are usually very ready. During the first few months of babymaking, most couples are relaxed and enjoy their relationship, anticipating that nature will take its course. They have every reason to be hopeful. But for one out of every six couples, the dream is transformed into a nightmare, and their hope becomes despair. Even when all the ingredients are seemingly present, pregnancy is not always the outcome.

Infertility is defined as the inability to conceive a child after a year or more of unprotected intercourse, or the inability to carry a pregnancy to a live birth. For those couples who come from particularly fertile families, or whose reproductive functioning has never been in question, infertility is usually a shock. Ironically, infertile women are often the ones who have had regular menstrual cycles, minimal cramps, and are otherwise in excellent health. Prior to their infertility they may never have seen a gynecologist for anything other than a routine check-up or a pap smear.

Some couples attempt conception anticipating infertility. The woman may have had gynecological problems in the past; she may have had infrequent or irregular menstrual periods. The man may have had an undescended testicle at birth, or a severe case of mumps. Perhaps a sibling had been infertile, or one of their mothers had had difficulty conceiving.

Many women who anticipate infertility do so because they have a history of being a Diethylstilbesterol (DES) daughter, or a Dalkon Shield user. Others have had previous abortions, or a sexually transmitted disease that might have caused Pelvic Inflammatory Disease. These women are usually filled with guilt about their histories. A diagnosis of infertility reminds them of past traumas and creates a new, though irrational, fear—that they are being punished for a previous sin. These women are not shocked by their infertility, yet they are still devastated.

Many couples today postpone childbearing until they have met certain goals such as establishing careers, purchasing homes, or traveling. Generally they are people who feel they have control over their lives, who believe that hard work and determination will produce desired results. Infertility is often the first disaster they encounter, the first time their life design did not progress according to the specs. These couples not only blame themselves, but they may also be blamed by family, friends, and even medical professionals for waiting so long to have children. Endometriosis, for example, is referred to as "the career woman's disease," as if it might easily have been avoided, if only the woman in question had been more "normal" and had not been determined to fulfill herself through work as well as through motherhood.

Some couples deny their infertility and wait months or even years before seeking out medical help. Perhaps the realization is too painful, even unthinkable. They may keep a tally of the number of menstrual cycles left before they turn thirty-five or forty, or whatever age after which they've decided it would be too late to have a child. But whenever they conclude there is a problem, the journey from bedroom to the doctor's office is a difficult one.

Whether expected or unexpected, the diagnosis and dawning realization of infertility is a severe blow. The fact that a couple may never be able to have biological children puts them in touch with their earliest feelings of rage, sadness, and helplessness. For the more "fortunate" infertile couples, this realization closely precedes a cure, but for many others, the struggle continues for many months and years, permeating their lives and wearing them down.

Infertile people feel isolated. Even though the problem is quite common, most couples feel alone, certain everyone else becomes pregnant easily. They probably know few, if any, other infertile couples. As they enter the bewildering maze of medical tests and procedures, they need companionship. Yet many go through it alone, sometimes feeling ashamed of their infertility. The most private aspect of their lives is now under medical scrutiny. It is difficult to share it with others, even with those who care.

This book attempts to diminish isolation. We have organized it into chapters that we feel address the main concerns of infertile couples, their families, and caregivers. We talk about diagnosis, treatment, emotional effects, and the impact of infertility on relationships, career, and religion. We talk about pregnancy loss, new and alternative reproductive technologies, secondary infertility, moving on, adoption, childfree living, and pregnancy and parenting after infertility. We have tried to provide the reader with a good deal of practical information, but because we also remember the need to share, we have involved many others in our project.

We bring you a selection of essays and poems about infertility written by both men and women. Some of these people are in the midst of diagnosis and treatment; others have long ago resolved their infertility. Some are mothers and fathers through birth or adoption; some are childfree. These writers have a variety of stories to tell and, as we hoped, they tell them in different voices—some sad, some humorous; all poignant.

In selecting essays to include, we have looked not only for a variety of experiences, but also for a variety of perspectives. Some chapters include several essays and other chapters include but one. The importance of a particular chapter, however, should not be measured by the number of essays or poems included in it. There were some subjects about which several people wrote, and others in which we received only one essay. And unfortunately, due to space limitations, we had to eliminate some very special pieces. All of the chapters are important; we could not possibly prioritize them. Together they encompass the range of the infertility experience as we see it.

Our authors include an infertility specialist, a rabbi, two psychiatrists, a baker, a lawyer, a minister, a musician, an elementary school principal. They come from various areas in the United States. We located them by advertising in RESOLVE newsletters, by word of mouth, and through our support groups. We contacted a friend last seen twenty years ago and strangers whose names we found in newspapers or magazines. Some of our authors are professional writers and others have never before written anything for publication. Some used their real names and others chose to use pseudonyms.

As we go to press in the spring of 1988, we are mindful of the changing nature of our subject matter. New problems are being diagnosed and new treatments recommended. We remember, for example, that a year-and-a-half ago, when we began this book, in vitro fertilization (IVF) and gamete intra-fallopian transfer (GIFT) were unusual procedures, reserved only for the most hopeless situations. Today, they are widely accepted treatments for a range of infertility problems. Adoption, too, is undergoing changes. Many adoptive parents are finding babies in nontraditional ways, and in many such situations, all members of the adoption triangle are exploring and acknowledging their interconnections in a more open way. Infertile couples have more choices and challenges than ever before.

We hope that this book fulfills its intended purpose: to offer guidance, support, and comfort. We hope that our readers will be soothed and inspired by the courage of others, many still struggling, many resolved. In addition, we hope that caregivers working in the field of infertility—physicians, their support staff, nurses, and psychotherapists—will also benefit from this book. The collective feelings, experiences, and wisdom of our fifty authors cannot help but enhance their empathy and understanding as it surely enhanced ours.

I Dream about Being Pregnant

Katherine Schneider Aker

I dream about being
pregnant, as if I did not know it could
not be, as if my sleeping mind is still
denying my infertility, my
sterility. Sometimes I think of
babies' names, as if there might yet be an
opportunity to sift through names until
finding just the right one for the perfect
baby, but when I am
awake, I catch myself, remind myself that it will
never be and that my
energy is better channeled elsewhere. I
no longer read articles written by
mothers of young children, but, with a little
surge of resentment, turn past them in
my magazines, appalled at the amount of
space they take up, and wondering if I should
cancel all my subscriptions. The whole
world seems in a conspiracy to keep my
self-pity alive; the newspapers,
crammed with updates on contraception; the
shopping malls, peopled with
pregnant women, glowing largely and
heel-walking everywhere, and
babies, like fat sausages, their skin so tight
around them. I cannot
touch them or speak to them, but must
ignore them, developing a kind of
selective sight while I try to
heal myself and accept what is without
driving myself into madness and
despair.

1

The Medical Work-Up
and Treatment

INFERTILITY, like any life crisis, creates emotional anguish for the individuals involved. But infertility, unlike some crises, is also a medical condition that requires physical, often painful, interventions. Test after test must be performed, each one having its own unique demands relative to scheduling, physical discomfort, and emotional distress. And because the woman is the potential childbearer, it is she who must undergo most of the physical pain.

Couples are usually advised to seek medical attention for infertility if they have not conceived after a year of unprotected sexual intercourse. Some couples, however, seek help after six months, and others may wait a few years before consulting a physician. No matter when they enter treatment, however, there are certain tests that must be included in a thorough work-up. Ideally, the couple should seek help from a qualified infertility specialist, or, if that is not possible, a gynecologist knowledgeable about infertility. When a problem is diagnosed and treated, the process is generally halted.

If the treatment does not eventually result in conception, the work-up proceeds accordingly. One of the dangers, though, in halting the work-up while a treatment is being tried, is that sometimes another, perhaps even more serious problem, is not discovered. Patients and their physicians must agree not to let too much time elapse before continuing their work-up when a particular treatment does not result in conception.

Most infertility work-ups begin with temperature charts. Women are told to take their temperature each morning using a basal body thermometer in order to determine when and if they are ovulating. Recent medical developments, such as Ovustick, allow the woman to determine, even more precisely, when she is ovulating, though ovulation predictors are used most effectively as adjuncts to basal body temperature monitoring. Always, basal body temperature must be taken before getting out of bed in the morning. This simple task may become monumentally difficult for some women, particularly after months or years of charts with peaks and valleys going nowhere. Occasionally, couples take breaks from temperature charting, but doctors usually require it, so the process is resumed. Sometimes, this morning routine becomes an obsession for couples, as well as a constant reminder of their pain.

In addition to charting daily temperature, the couple must also indicate when they had sexual relations, in order to determine whether they are "hitting" optimal days. A circle around a particular day indicates coitus. The most private aspect of their lives thus becomes public record. Many couples, eventually confess "fudging" some of their circles, lest their doctor think they are not really interested in having a child.

Women are used to being poked and prodded; that is the nature of the gynecological exam. Familiarity, however, does not mean complacency, especially when the tests are extremely uncomfortable and almost always invasive. Some of the embarrassment at being naked with one's feet in stirrups diminishes with time, but the sense of helplessness and vulnerability persists as the work-up (and later treatment) progresses.

One of the more painful procedures a woman undergoes is the endometrial biopsy, in which a piece of uterine lining is scraped off and examined just prior to menstruation. The purpose of this test is to determine whether the woman has ovulated properly, and whether the endometrium (lining of the uterus) is of sufficient quality for an embryo to implant itself. The biopsy does not take very long, but it can be quite painful; some women need medication to dull the physical sensations during the ordeal, though other women report feeling minimal pain.

Another standard part of the infertility work-up, and an even more painful procedure, is the hysterosalpingogram (tubogram) in which dye is inserted through the cervix into the uterus. The dye then travels into the fallopian tubes. The purpose of this test is to determine whether the tubes are open. If the dye does not make it through the tubes, then there is a blockage somewhere. In order to perform the tubogram a canula is inserted into the cervical canal and the cervix is pulled tightly onto it. Sometimes this is done by attaching a suction cup to the woman's cervix. The pain can be excruciating. But, like the endometrial biopsy, women experience the tubogram very differently. One woman claimed that it was "no worse than having a tooth filled," while another woman described the procedure by saying "it felt like my insides were being pulled out of me."

A laparoscopy is another important diagnostic tool in an infertility work-up. This surgical procedure must be performed under general anesthesia, and is therefore more risky and often more anxiety provoking than other tests. In a laparoscopy, a small incision is made through the navel, and a laparoscope inserted. The physician looks for endometriosis, adhesions, or any other structural abnormalities that might prevent conception or implantation. Women can actually see the X-ray results of their uterus and tubes, and many report feeling relieved when seeing a normal reproductive system. Some women, however, are afraid of general anesthesia, and their reservations about the procedure reflect their fears about losing control, or about possible complications from the anesthesia. Other women are relieved to be "put to sleep," secure in the knowledge that they will feel no pain. Though the laparoscopy itself is a one-day outpatient operation, recuperation often takes a few additional days.

Some tests, though less painful or risky, are inconvenient, as they must be timed precisely, and thus usually interfere with one's job, social life, and marital or sexual relationship. One such test, requiring cooperation of both husband and wife, is the post-coital (PK) exam, in which a sample of cervical mucus is taken within a few hours of having sexual intercourse. The PK test indicates whether a sufficient number of healthy sperm are able to penetrate the cervical mucus and make swift forward progress. This test often requires that the couple have intercourse early in the morning on a working day, a time many find is not conducive to sexual relations.

There are other tests in an infertility work-up that require cooperation between husband and wife. These include testing for mycoplasma and chlamydia, organisms that are a cross between a virus and bacteria, and are passed back and forth between a couple. Testing involves obtaining a cervical mucus culture from the woman, and a urine culture from the man. Treatment for these virus/bacterium involves taking an antibiotic such as Tetracycline for about ten days. It is essential that both members of the couple be recultured, as both mycoplasma and chlamydia are sometimes resistant to certain antibiotics. An absolute connection between infertility and these virus/bacterium has not been determined. Some physicians are therefore reluctant to test for them, claiming that many women who have given birth test positively for mycoplasma or chlamydia. Research, however, seems to indicate that when they are found and treated in infertile women, a greater percentage go on to conceive than would be expected by chance.

Testing for antibodies is another important part of an infertility work-up. There are two possible types of antibodies that can be causes of infertility.

The first type may be present in the woman's cervical mucus, and therefore would kill any sperm. Testing for this involves obtaining a sample of cervical mucus from the woman twenty-four hours after intercourse, as well as a blood sample. The test is performed about midcycle. The second type of antibodies that may be found are antibodies that a man has to his own sperm. This can be measured by drawing a blood sample from him.

Couples have sexual relations feeling, to some degree, that the doctor is in the bedroom with them, checking on their performance. Sometimes men become impotent when faced with this pressure, or they have difficulty ejaculating. Their wives become frustrated, adding extra tension to an already highly charged situation. Scheduled intercourse, for procreation or diagnosis, often becomes the root of marital conflict. Many couples report that one of them can generally be counted on to begin an argument that is sometimes so alienating, intercourse is neither possible nor desired.

The male infertility work-up is medically simple. It consists of a general check-up including a scrotal examination. The physician is searching for a varicocele (a varicose vein in the scrotum) that might be a possible cause of male infertility. The male infertility work-up is not painful, but it involves producing a sperm sample, about which most men get embarrassed. Although the sample can be produced at home, most doctors prefer it be done at their office. The man must go into a men's room (or a neighboring office), masturbate, and ejaculate into a jar. His sperm are then analyzed for count, motility, and morphology (shape). If everything is within normal range, he probably won't have to go back, at least not for a sperm analysis, for some time. If the results are inconclusive, or below normal, this will probably be the first of many samples he will be asked to produce.

Most males learned to be secretive about masturbation when they were adolescents. The notion of having to be public about this usually furtive act is extremely embarrassing. Men dread the idea of other people, including office staff and lab technicians, knowing what they are doing in the men's room. Even the most stable men end up feeling like insecure adolescents as a result of this procedure. They may also feel as if their masculinity is at stake.

Most couples undergoing an infertility work-up have mixed feelings about the results of the tests they take. On the one hand, they usually experience relief if no problem is detected. On the other hand, they feel new hope if a treatable problem is diagnosed. Depending on the medical diagnosis, and on the treatment options available, couples may or may not be relieved to have a particular problem. Some conditions, such as endometriosis, take several months to cure, precious time during which a couple must refrain from attempting to conceive.

Thirty years ago most infertile couples had one option: to adopt. They lived in a time when little was known about infertility and even less was available in the way of treatment. Their situation was difficult, in part, because they had so little control over it.

Times have changed. Recent advances in the diagnosis and treatment of infertility have presented many infertile couples with a range of options. They may be able to take medication, have surgery, or possibly try a combined approach. Couples are called upon to make decisions about their treatment every step along the way. However, even though there is a good chance that one treatment or another will work, the road to pregnancy may be difficult, uncertain, and in the end, prove fruitless.

Because the field of infertility is relatively new, and there are still many unanswered questions, there are many different opinions in the medical community regarding diagnosis and treatment. It is essential therefore, that a couple be as knowledgeable as possible about all aspects of their condition. Ultimately, it is they who must decide what treatment to pursue, or whether to seek another opinion. But no matter what viewpoint the doctor holds, or what treatment he or she recommends, the available options always fall within the same broad range of categories. These options involve decisions about medications, surgery, and alternative reproductive technologies. Each of these involves consideration of many factors, including risk, side effects, physical discomfort, and expenditures of time and money. Rather than attempting to discuss, within this brief introduction, the range of treatment options available to infertile couples, we have chosen instead to concentrate on the types of decisions that face the infertile couple as they travel down this difficult road.

Decisions about Medication

The first question that most infertility patients raise regarding medication has to do with safety. Having grown up in the shadow of DES, a drug once believed to be safe, now known to produce serious long-term side effects, infertility patients know that one cannot always predict whether a particular medication will ultimately harm them. Because most fertility drugs were developed within the past thirty years, no long-term studies of their effects have been done. Anyone electing to take a fertility drug is accepting some risk.

Infertility patients must deal with this risk factor by learning about a particular medication before deciding whether to take it. They need to ask their physicians about potential problems and read all they can about the drug. If they do decide to try it, they need to pay close attention to their bodies. Some people do decide not to take drugs, perhaps because of some past personal or family problem with medication, or personal convictions about drugs. But most accept the risks involved and conclude that the potential gain outweighs them.

Closely related to the issue of risk, is the problem of side effects. Patients need to consider the "wear and tear" on their physical and emotional selves in taking fertility medications. For example, some patients complain of weight gain, visual problems, or depression while taking clomiphene. Most, however, find that taking this medication—usually one or two tablets for five to seven days—is a relatively simple regimen. Few patients will elect not to take clomiphene on the basis of side effects or difficulties in the treatment protocol.

Danocrine (Danazol), the medication most often prescribed for the pharmacological treatment of endometriosis, poses greater problems. Patients are often troubled by the weight gain, skin changes, and masculinizing side effects of the medication. They are also bothered by the treatment regimen that often requires several well-timed doses daily for six or more months. Pergonal, the "big gun" of fertility drugs, is powerful enough to cause ovarian hyperstimulation, a serious and potentially life threatening condition. Most often, close medical supervision can avoid or correct this condition. But patients must also consider how they feel about multiple births since this is something that can be watched, but not necessarily prevented.

Pergonal also presents patients with a different sort of challenge. Unlike patients with endometriosis, who must wait at least six months to see if their medication worked, Pergonal patients are involved in an intense drama each month. Most are given their daily injections at a precise time of day, often administered by their husbands. The injections are followed up with blood tests and ultrasounds. Patients taking Pergonal watch their estrogen rise and their follicles grow, awaiting the time when a single injection of human chorionic gonadotropin (HCG) will trigger ovulation. They keep a close eye on the action while tension mounts.

The issue of efficacy is also an important one in considering medication. Couples want a drug that will work, and it is their faith in the drug's potential that enables them to commit the time, energy, and money involved. Patients soon learn, however, that medications vary in their effectiveness from person to person and often, from cycle to cycle. Hence it is frequently necessary to change or alter treatment regimens. This situation is most common in the treatment of ovulatory problems. Some patients conceive on fifty milligrams of clomiphene, while others need a higher dose. For some, it is the combination of clomiphene and progesterone that works. And still other women require Pergonal in order to ovulate.

In considering medications, infertility patients must also consider the cost. All fertility medications are expensive, but some far more so than others. While many insurance plans cover part or all of the cost of medications, some do not. Pergonal, for example, can run into several hundred dollars per cycle, a cost that cannot be ignored. For many patients, the price will limit whether, and for how long, they can take the medication.

Decisions about Surgery

Infertility patients usually make decisions about surgery more actively, and with more conflict, than decisions about medication. While they are sensitive to the risks involved in taking drugs, there is something more dramatic—and more threatening—about surgery. With medication, the question is usually what to take, and for how long. With surgery, people often have serious reservations about undergoing the procedure at all since it means subjecting themselves to general anesthesia, physical discomfort, and a long convalescence, in addition to the risks involved.

People elect surgery in order to have something fixed. Infertility patients learn quickly though, that fixing a problem does not necessarily mean pregnancy. A man can have his varicocele repaired, see an improvement in his sperm count, and still fail to impregnate his wife. A woman can have her endometriosis surgically removed, but still not conceive. And worse still, is the woman who undergoes a tubal repair only to end up with an ectopic pregnancy months later.

In considering surgery, patients usually look more carefully at statistics. They want the odds to be in their favor. A 30 percent rate of cure with medication probably sounds better than a 30 percent cure with major surgery. On the other hand, many patients are told that without surgery, conception is not possible. They often feel compelled to gamble no matter what the odds are.

Decisions Regarding the New Reproductive Technologies

The decision to try one of the new reproductive technologies—in vitro fertilization (IVF) or gamete intra fallopian transfer (GIFT)—is especially complex. Not only do these procedures involve taking powerful medications and undergoing surgery, but they are also very expensive, rarely being covered by insurance. In addition, the procedures are time consuming, extremely stressful, and offer little chance of success. In a later chapter we will discuss the new reproductive technologies more thoroughly, including all the complexities of decision making.

In working with infertile couples, we try to help them make informed, well thought out decisions. We support their efforts to educate themselves, to ask questions of their physicians, and to talk together about what makes sense for them as a couple. When they disagree about timing, or about the choice of treatment, we try to help them listen to each other and to respond to their partner's feelings as well as their own.

Sometimes we come across individuals and couples who make decisions with which we do not agree. We are surprised that some will continue to try a treatment that has not worked, while others will turn down a promising option. We have learned that we can help people to have accurate information, but they must make their own decisions about this highly personal matter. Some are determined to try every available treatment, while others identify clear limits to what they are prepared to do physically, emotionally, and financially.

In the following pages we offer four essays: two on the medical work-up and two on treatment. Ellen Jean Tepper and Larry Cooper recount, with humor, incidents that were part of their infertility work-up: the post-coital (PK) test and the sperm sample. Though infertility itself is nothing to laugh about, most couples find that it does help to maintain a sense of humor about their predicament. Alexis Brown offers a brief account of her experience with endometriosis, a medical condition that can be physically painful as well as cause infertility. And finally, Carmella Horlitz discusses her experience taking Pergonal, a powerful fertility drug that can, in some instances, cause serious side effects—or delightful ones—in her case, twins.

PK

Ellen Jean Tepper

Of PK tests, I have known many. Poor ones, worse ones, invalid ones, and, at long last, the mediocre.

I came upon my first PK test rather innocently. For a year or so I had been treated for ovulatory problems with Clomid. But no pregnancy had resulted and my doctor, Dr. P, and I had both begun to wonder whether there were other factors affecting my fertility. He'd suggested another series of tests, one of them being the PK.

Dr. P's instructions were simple enough. Dave and I were to "abstain" for two days prior to the test. Then, between seven and eight A.M. on the appointed morning, we were to have "relations." I was to go directly to Dr. P's office.

"Are you sure that you had relations this morning?" Dr. P looked puzzled when he returned from the microscope.

Needless to say, I was sure. At least I was sure that that morning we had done what we had been doing together for thirteen years. I worried, for a moment, that we had been doing it wrong all this time. Then I wondered more seriously about the brisk walk that I'd taken when I found I had a few minutes to spare.

"Dr. P, do you think that they fell out on my way over? Maybe I shouldn't have gone for a walk after having sex?" (I hoped he wouldn't mind my using the word sex.) He assured me that sperm don't simply fall out of vaginas, but added that he had no explanation for where they were. Even if there was a problem, he explained, we'd see lots of dead sperm. The fact that there were none was truly a mystery. I could tell that he was still wondering whether we'd really had sex.

Dr. P recommended that we give the sperm forty-eight hours to re-group and try again.

"You move too fast. You must have dropped them out on the way over." That was Dave's response. I was careful not to tell him about the walk. "Just move slowly next time and things will be fine."

I approached my second PK test cautiously. I drove slowly, kept my legs pressed together, and waddled into the office. I avoided urinating, fearful that the sperm would land in Dr. P's toilet. This time I had done it right.

Dr. P returned from the microscope. He looked somber. "There are sperm there, but this time they are all dead."

My third and fourth PK tests occurred one month later. Dr. P had suggested that we plan two tests, spaced forty-eight hours apart. The first would repeat what we had done, hopefully with different results. "Maybe it was just a bad month?" Dr. P posited. "Sometimes sperm production is compromised by an infection or a virus." But he went on to suggest that we try husband insemination if there was another bad test.

PK test no. 3 was a repeat of the first. No walk. No peeing. Still no sperm, living or dead. Test no. 4 was to fall on Rosh Hashanah, the Jewish New Year.

"You mean that we're going to have to leave temple early so that I can jerk off into a jar in your doctor's office?" Dave was hardly enchanted with the idea.

The Rosh Hashanah service is a celebration of fertility. The Torah portion talks about Sarah, so long barren, who finally gave birth. I was lost in some thoughts about her fertility, and that of her "sisters," Leah and Rachel, when Dave commented, "I guess Mary was the only one in the Bible without a fertility problem." It was time to go.

So Dr. P celebrated his New Year and we celebrated ours standing over the microscope, looking for live sperm. There were none.

"Well, I guess there is something seriously wrong with the sperm. They look normal but they self-destruct."

"They self-destruct or they're being destroyed by the mucus?" I wondered why Dr. P was blaming it on the sperm? While I kind of liked the idea that I was not the only one with a problem, I couldn't follow his reasoning. Dave's sperm had passed several laboratory evaluations with flying colors. My fertility, by contrast, had little to recommend it. "Dr. P, why don't you inseminate me with donor sperm and see how they do?"

"But you could become pregnant!"

I was willing to take my chances on that one.

PK test no. 5. This time I wasn't sure how I wanted things to turn out. If it was bad, then it confirmed my fear that there was something inexplicably wrong with my mucus. I didn't like that idea, but there was some advantage to having only one patient in the family. If the donor sperm fared well then Dave too was implicated. We would have two specialists, possibly two treatment regimes. We might find ourselves in the unexpected and difficult position of having to consider donor insemination seriously.

"Well, I was right," pronounced Dr. P "The problem is with the sperm. This PK test with donor sperm is fine."

"Really?" I was stunned. "Are there lots of live sperm? And can they really swim?"

"No, I found two and they are both moving."

"But I thought that anything less than five was a very poor test."

"One is all it takes." Dr. P declared. "Dave, I think it's time for you to see a specialist."

Dave agreed to this recommendation. I left the office that day convinced that two out of three people were crazy and that I wasn't one of them.

What followed was a negative work-up by Dr. K, the urologist that Dr. P had recommended. Dr. K's findings supported the results of all the earlier semen analyses. Dave's sperm were plentiful, of good quality, with excellent motility. He confirmed what I'd known all along.

"I'm afraid that Dr. K is missing something. Those sperm are simply not normal."

"But Dr. P," I tried to reason, "The donor sperm died too. You are placing a lot of faith in those two little buggers that managed to survive my attack mucus. I'd rather put my faith in Dr. K's lab."

We were clearly at a stalemate.

I was preparing to seek a second opinion when my mother-in-law's latest mailing on infertility arrived. These dispatches had been coming about once a month for the past four years. I knew that she meant well but had tired of hearing about the doctor in Bangor, Maine, who had cured her cousin's best friend's niece, or the recipe for warm rum and milk that was sure to relax the uterus at bedtime.

"Arm and Hammer is the Latest Fertility Drug." The headline caught my eye and I read on. "Women whose cervical mucus is too acidic can establish a more hospitable environment by douching with baking soda and warm water one-half hour before intercourse." The clipping was from *Parade* magazine. Still, I was willing to give it a try.

"You can believe in black magic if you want, but the truth is that your husband has a serious fertility problem. The two of you cannot have a child together."

At this point, I figured that I had two choices. I could go out and find another infertility specialist, wait a few months for an appointment, and then another week or so for a PK test. Or I could figure out a way to get someone else in Dr. P's office to do the test.

"Hello, I need to make an appointment for my husband and me to talk with Dr. P. I'll need to confirm a time with Dave, but wanted to find out which days Dr. P is available."

"He's in the office every day but Wednesday and Friday mornings when he's in the operating room. Also, he'll be out of town for two weeks beginning on the sixteenth."

There I had it. My mucus would be optimal for a few days during Dr. P's vacation.

My sixth PK test was done by Dr. M, a young man who must have been doing a fellowship with Dr. P. He came upon me innocently, unaware that he was soon to bring Dave's sperm back from death row. "I hear that you've come for a PK test."

"Yes," I interrupted, not wanting him to have a chance to say that I didn't need another. "Yes, I haven't done too well on them in the past, but I want to give it one last try. And today I'm prepared to pay five dollars for every live sperm you can find." Dr. M laughed. Then he took the specimen and headed for the microscope. Moments later I heard him calling.

"Come quick! Look! You owe me a lot of money." And there they were. Not an army, but about five or six live sperm. "They look great. They are swimming freely!" Dr. M was ready to take out the champagne.

When Dr. P heard the news, he said that Dr. M was seeing things. I was tempted to argue, to prove my point with another PK. Instead, I got a refill of my Clomid and invested in another large box of baking soda.

As it turned out, two tablespoons was all I needed.

The Sperm Sample
Larry Cooper

A strong desire to become a father got me through my male infertility work-up. Before hand, I had no idea how awkward and embarrassing a "medical" procedure could be. Looking back now, as the father of two, I can laugh, but at the time I found very little humor in it all.

I approached the office with trepidation, focusing on my genitals, figuring they would be the only part of me in which the doctor was interested. Sure enough, his exam began with a scrotal feel (probably not the technical name) and moved on to questions about frequency and position of intercourse. I tried to act calm and cool as I answered him. Then he told me to make an appointment for a semen analysis.

As the day of reckoning approached, I wondered what the procedure would be like. Would there be a dimly lit room showing stag films? A soft couch with a supply of *Playboy* magazines? A nice looking, well-endowed nurse to help me out if I needed it? No such luck!

My initial worry was that there would be a crowded elevator and everyone on it would know where I was going and what I was going to do. The lab, however, was located in a remote research building, part of the Harvard teaching hospital where our specialist worked. There was no one on the elevator, and as I approached the lab, the corridor was clear. I began to wonder if this was an unusual event. I imagined that the staff would be talking about me for days.

The lab itself was reminiscent of my high school chemistry class. There were tables filled with test tubes, beakers, and Petri dishes. I wondered whether these vessels were full of billions of unrequited sperm, and I wondered how mine would fare among them. Within just a few minutes, my fantasies had gone from the unusual to the ordinary.

I cleared my throat so that one of the lab technicians would know that I had arrived. In fact she had been expecting me. I could not decide whether this was evidence for the unusual or the ordinary theory. I was handed a jar and told to go down the hall to the men's room and deposit a sample in the jar. As I walked to the lavatory, I wondered how this would work. Was the men's room that special environment of my fantasies, or was this two-inch deep glass jar to be my only companion?

Again I was taken back in time—to junior high school—the men's room reminded me of the boys' room in that seventy-year-old institution. The only fixtures were a sink with a mirror above it, a urinal, and a single enclosed toilet stall. I looked around and laughed. My pleasurable fantasies had turned into a joke on me! I decided to be mature about the situation. I looked at the jar and said to myself, "Let's get this over with." Since the men's room door did not lock, I decided that the enclosed toilet stall was the only possible place for this rendezvous with myself. I wondered how many men had masturbated here before me. Had those with poor aim somehow left their mark? Fortunately, the stall did lock but I worried that someone might decide to use the urinal while I was trying to fill the jar. I feared I would be distracted in my mission.

Since it was winter, I removed my overcoat, but there was no place to hang it. I draped it over the stall wall, doing the same with my sport jacket. But what if someone came in and recognized my clothing? Just as I was thinking that I should have come in disguise, I noticed the worst. The toilet had no cover. I would either have to sit on the open toilet seat as though I were using it for its intended purpose, or I would have to stand up. After trying both, I decided that standing up would give me a better shot at hitting the target.

Fortunately, my fears of being impotent with a glass jar proved unfounded. As I took aim and fired, I remembered what it felt like to be an awkward adolescent, masturbating quietly on the other side of my parents' bedroom wall, praying I would not be discovered. I did hit the target, and returned triumphantly to the lab. As I held the jar up proudly I felt the earth cave in under my feet, as the lab attendant exclaimed, "Oh, back so soon!"

Endometriosis

Alexis Brown

My period began when I was fifteen. At that time, I was so relieved to finally be "like everybody else" that I took the pain in stride. I saw other girls going about their normal activities when they had "their friend" and assumed that they handled cramps better than I did. And as I sat doubled over on the side lines at gym, I figured that my mother and others were right when they suggested that I'd found a handy way out of my worst subject.

For the next eight years, I continued to accept my monthly torture as the norm. If there was a problem, it was my pain threshold. Then, when I was twenty-two, I developed severe abdominal pain and was admitted for emergency surgery. When I awoke my misery had a name.

Endometriosis. At first I was pleased to have an explanation. I had been terrified before the surgery and so I was relieved to awaken and learn that I had a chronic disease and not a terminal illness. When my doctor explained further what was happening—that blood was spilling into the uterine cavity, around the bowels and alongside my ovaries—I felt vindicated. No wonder I'd had such a hard time with my periods!

What I did not understand at the time of diagnosis was that endometriosis meant more than painful periods. In many cases, and mine is one, it means infertility as well. But at twenty-two and single, I was not thinking about my ability to bear children. And the doctors didn't answer questions that I didn't ask.

When I was twenty-six, I needed more surgery. The endometriosis that had been treated four years earlier was back and was again causing severe abdominal pain. But this time I was concerned with more than my immediate suffering. I'd met the man that I wanted to marry and we were eager to start a family.

I had a second laporatomy during our first year of marriage. To further maximize my chances to conceive, I took a six-month course of Danocrine, a male hormone that suppresses the monthly cycle. The idea is that it will shrink the endometriosis. The problem is that there are side effects: weight gain, mood changes, headaches. Worse yet, it meant six months with no chance of conception.

Had the surgeries and the Danocrine led to a pregnancy, I would surely look back and say that it was all worth it. But they did not. I am thirty and childless, trying to hold on to hope, as it grows dim.

Often, I think back on the fifteen year old who was so delighted to be menstruating. In my innocence, I regarded my painful periods as necessary, as the price I had to pay for the rights and privileges of being a woman. Central among these was the right to reproduce.

My endometriosis presents a serious challenge to that right. Nature's well-designed system has gone haywire.

Pergonal:
The Final Step
Carmela Horlitz

Our careers were going well. Yet at thirty years old, confronting our mortality and our ten-year marriage, we wanted a sense of home and family of our own. We decided to have children. After two years without a pregnancy, we sought medical treatment.

We were used to having some control over our destiny; of succeeding at whatever we put our minds to. But here, we worked and worked at a problem and could see no progress. At the beginning of our infertility evaluation, I started seeing a counselor and, somehow, began coping better. Our families were very supportive of our struggle and that helped ease the pain, except for holidays.

Our infertility evaluation gave us a clean slate. We were "normal" infertiles, although there was some indication that I might be experiencing some luteal phase problems, that is, inadequate progestrone secretion after ovulation, which interferes with implantation and pregnancy. So I began Clomid therapy for nine cycles, and saw another three-quarters of a year go by. Once again, I was told that I could get pregnant any time.

The next step was a big one—Pergonal. I had heard of the rigors and the side effects of this treatment—as well as the multiple births—and was frightened to try it. But we were at the end of the line, so there wasn't much of a choice. I was nearly thirty-five and I wanted a baby.

Each Pergonal program follows a slightly different protocol. My experience was one in which a group of patients would all start Pergonal on the same day. An infertility specialist oversaw the program with assistance from nurse practitioners or medical residents who followed patients individually, consulted with the specialist daily, and dealt with each patient's multiple questions and concerns.

As I had anticipated, taking Pergonal was a time-consuming and stressful experience. I spent a good deal of time running from one area of the hospital to another—for a pelvic exam, blood work, and an ultrasound. The cost of the medication *alone* was about forty dollars a day.

I am a nurse so I am comfortable with preparing medication. But preparing injections is very different from giving them to yourself! I learned to inject myself in the thighs, but the process was a painful one. Then there was the issue of privacy and my job. I had a wonderful supportive woman as my boss. We worked, however, in a somewhat sexist environment. I had a terrible time keeping my infertility problem as private as possible, and trying not to let my emotions interfere with my job performance. I tried very hard, but I m sure I wasn't nearly as successful as I wanted to be. I realized later that I'd vented much of my anger about my infertility at my job and workplace. I seriously considered resigning, but felt I would become even more obsessed with infertility if I did.

In any event, I continued with both my job and Pergonal, making daily trips to Boston, about forty minutes each way, until I ovulated, then back about seven days later for bloodwork. Then I had to wait until my cycle began again . . . or I became pregnant. Of course, it also meant making love every other day around my anticipated time of ovulation. In addition, one or two PK tests were required each cycle. All of it was becoming tiresome. Fortunately, I never needed more than seven or eight days of Pergonal. And fortunately also, our insurance was excellent, covering 80 percent or more of the program, which was costing about $1500 per cycle. The money, however, was not an issue for us. We would have paid whatever we had to in order to conceive.

My first Pergonal cycle was unsuccessful in that I did not conceive. I did, however, respond favorably to the treatment, and was able to handle it physically and emotionally. We were encouraged and ready to try again, waiting a month to give my ovaries and veins a rest.

My next period was due on Thanksgiving Day, so my husband and I planned a quiet holiday together. By the Sunday after Thanksgiving, I still had no period and decided to have a pregnancy test the next day. I awoke Monday, feeling awful, my temperature had dropped and my period begun. But I had unusual cramping and a heavy flow. It was a very difficult day, during which I had trouble controlling my emotions. Its memory remains strong now, five years later. Although it was not documented, the doctor felt that I was probably pregnant and had miscarried. I cannot say that this early loss of pregnancy made it any easier or any less real than had I been pregnant two months or more. It really hurt.

Soon after the pregnancy loss, I learned that a friend had become pregnant on Pergonal. Perhaps irrationally, because I hoped his "magic" would work with me, I decided to change to her doctor. His program required daily bloodwork throughout the cycle, with an ultrasound and exams every five days until ovulation, and post-coital exams just prior to ovulation. My husband, an electrical engineer, really liked this program. He coped with the stress of infertility by thriving on more data, and this program supplied a multitude of data. My husband drew my bloods so I only had to drop off bloods every five days once I passed ovulation, thus reducing time away from work. He also learned to administer injections in my buttocks and give me the Pergonal, as well as assuming responsibility for recording my temperature on the chart. All these things lightened the burden of Pergonal immensely, and allowed me some relief from its intense responsibility.

I completed this cycle, failed to conceive, and felt ready to terminate treatment. I wanted to get on with my life. However, my husband was not ready to quit and I agreed to try again.

I am a Roman Catholic and I decided to attend a Healing Service as a means of resolving my infertility. I hoped, first, that it would heal my mind and heart, but I must admit that I secretly hoped it would cure me of my infertility as well. I attended the service with my husband and found that it did help a great deal. We prayed and cried together, and emerged feeling relieved. We felt prepared to go on with Pergonal, but were also accepting of our next option—adoption.

My next Pergonal cycle did not go smoothly. I required extra doses of the medication because I was developing several small follicles rather than one or two dominant follicles that could ripen. The first post-coital exam was very bad; the slide was covered with dead sperm. I kept reminding myself that this was not my fault, I couldn't control these things. Somehow it did help. The next post-coital the following day was good. I ovulated. It was Easter Sunday, spring, time for rebirth.

My period was due on a Monday, so we took a trip over the weekend to keep busy. I had no symptoms at all. By Friday, I had no period, but I felt as if I had the flu. I decided to wait until Monday to take a pregnancy test. The flu was going around so I thought it was the cause of my delayed period and my symptoms. I dared not hope otherwise. I called the doctor's office early Tuesday for the pregnancy test results and it was positive! The numerical value of the beta subunit was very high. The nurse advised me to find an obstetrician as soon as possible and call her back in a week. I could hardly contain myself. I called my husband at work as we had arranged. We were almost afraid to believe it was happening. After my first obstetrical visit three weeks later, we made the news public. I was only two months pregnant, very symptomatic, eating constantly, and very, very tired.

At about eleven weeks pregnant, I returned to the Pergonal program for an ultrasound—"to check things out," according to the nurse. The same technician and radiologist who had done many of my other ultrasounds were there, as was my husband. Together, we saw the real miracle: two hearts beating on the screen at the same time. There was no doubt about it—twins. We were shocked but happy. Although we knew the odds of having multiple births from Pergonal is about 20 percent, we never really believed it possible for us. On reflection, I did recall that the final ultrasound during the cycle indicated that I had two follicles about to ripen, but since I'd faced so many other failures, I gave it little thought. It took some getting used to, but we were excited.

I enjoyed a wonderful pregnancy with minimal problems. I felt much less concerned than I thought I would, but my husband was very protective of me and this pregnancy. I stopped working at thirty-two weeks and delivered three weeks later: a boy, Karl, four pounds fourteen ounces and a girl, Katherine, three pounds fifteen ounces. They were premature, very tiny, but okay.

Our children are four years old now, and they remain precious to us. I am very involved with them and most of the time I enjoy being a full-time mother. Still, I think about my infertility often and remain concerned for those who now travel that difficult road. Though blessed with a wonderful outcome, I will not forget the journey.

2
The Doctor-Patient Relationship

PERHAPS no area of medicine calls for collaboration between physician and patient as much as does the diagnosis and treatment of infertility. From temperature charts to Pergonal shots, infertility patients must participate actively in their own care. And, in the best of circumstances, this collaborative effort makes the experience easier for both physician and patient, since it gives the physician needed information and assistance, and offers the patient the opportunity to regain some sense of control.

Unfortunately, all infertility patients do not feel that they have a smooth working relationship with their doctor. Traditionally, patients have been viewed as sick, the physician as healthy. The former naive, the latter omnipotent. The physician more often male, the patient female. Unfortunately, this stereotype only serves to increase patients' anxiety about going to doctor's appointments, and prevents them from viewing themselves as equals, and asserting their rights as consumers.

Making the initial appointment to see an infertility specialist is often the hardest step for a couple. It means confronting their problem — dealing with it, and feeling the pain. And, since couples feel very vulnerable exposing the most intimate aspect of their lives to a stranger, it is no wonder that many wait months and even years longer than they should, before seeking medical help. Furthermore, most women probably have an already established relationship with a gynecologist whom they are reluctant to leave.

Most infertility patients are in a great deal of stress about their situation. Unfortunately, some physicians, though they may intellectually understand this, do not appear to be sensitive to the couple's feelings. When the couple do not feel that their physician empathizes with their struggle, they are far more reluctant to be open, to raise questions about their diagnosis and treatment, and to be partners with their physician, all of which are important ingredients in their treatment.

Certain kinds of situations and interactions in the physician's office enable the patient to feel well taken care of, while other situations contribute to the opposite feeling. The following are some of the areas that patients have identified as being most important.

Punctuality. It is important for your physician to be on time for your appointments. Doctors have emergencies and occasionally must be late, but patients who continually find themselves waiting for long periods of time before seeing the doctor have a right to feel angry and neglected. Doctors who schedule patients so that they are seen on time, and not rushed, are easier to have a good relationship with. These doctors put themselves on an equal basis with their patients, implying that the latter's time is as important as their own.

Undivided Attention. It is essential that you feel your physician is giving undivided attention to you during your office visit. Some patients report that their doctors often have many interruptions during their visit. Some doctors take phone calls; some have several examining rooms and go back and forth among them; and still others seem to get lost in paperwork. Doctors have been known to "forget" about their patients. For example, patients have complained about being left in examining rooms for extended periods of time with their feet in the stirrups. More sensitive doctors, however, are truly attentive. Interruptions are kept to a minimum, and their patients feel they are the focus of attention and that they are being listened to. These doctors (or their nurses) periodically check in on their patients if they are waiting for a procedure to be performed, or for the results of a certain test.

Time Allotment. It is essential that doctors spend enough time with their infertility patients. Some doctors rush their patients, giving explanations or directions with one foot out the door, or they hurriedly answer questions. With such a doctor, it's easy to feel minimized. Or to feel frustrated, leaving the doctor's office confused, and with unanswered questions. The most accessible doctors arrange their schedules so that they have enough time to answer questions thoroughly, and to offer any explanations or information that might be helpful to patients. Their patients leave the office feeling that their doctor is working with them in an orderly and sensible way, toward diagnosis and treatment.

Respect. Physicians must treat their patients as intelligent mature adults. Too often, doctors, perhaps in an effort to be comforting, sound patronizing, talking to their patients as if they were children. Often they call their patients by their first name, yet do not invite them to do likewise. People who ordinarily function competently and professionally in the world can easily feel dumb and insecure in such a doctor's presence. Look for a physician who addresses patients on an equal basis, offering clear, thorough explanations, though not in a demeaning manner. The idea is to feel like a collaborator with your doctor, not an underling.

Adequate Preparation. Infertility specialists must prepare their patients adequately for the procedures and tests they may undergo. Too often, women emerge from a hysterosalpingogram or other painful test, visibly shaken up. Their doctor had not told them how uncomfortable it might be, and they were unprepared for the degree of pain they felt. The more accessible doctors make sure they explain in detail everything a patient must do or that will be done to him or her. One patient said she was convinced that her endometrial biopsy was less painful because her doctor "walked" her through it. He would say soothingly, "Now you'll feel a little pull, next there will be a strong tug, now a scrape," etc. The more patients are prepared, not just for diagnostic tests, but also for possible treatment options, the better able they are to make informed choices about their treatment.

Support Staff. Perhaps most important, the infertility specialist's support staff, particularly nurses and secretaries, must be caring, sensitive people who understand the emotional strain that inevitably accompanies infertility. The manner and responses of nurses and/or secretaries can positively or negatively influence your experience. Many patients have been troubled by a lack of sensitivity and discretion. They refer to nurses who announce in front of a full waiting room, "Oh, you're here for your insemination," or who tell men they can use a baby food jar in which to collect their sperm sample. Look for a physician with support staff who show understanding and concern: the nurse who spends a few extra minutes in the examining room talking to a patient, or the secretary who goes out of her way to make sure the doctor quickly telephones back a worried patient.

Even in the best situations, the doctor-patient relationship can be stressful. Doctors are human. They make mistakes. They are busy. On the other hand, patients, though realistic, hope for miracles. The physician embodies that hope, and thus patients are often reluctant to do or say anything that might anger the doctor. Yet holding back from asking questions or from being critical only creates more of a gulf between patient and doctor.

We hope that the following guidelines will help in creating a truly positive, collaborative relationship between you and your doctor:

1. Remember that you are the employer. You hire the physician because he or she has certain expertise that you need. If you are not satisfied, you can fire the doctor and employ another.

2. You must educate yourself thoroughly about all aspects of infertility and reproductive medicine. No matter how skilled or how compulsive about record keeping the physician is, it should be remembered that he or she probably has well over a hundred patients, perhaps many more. Mistakes can be made. Facts can be forgotten. When there is only one patient—yourself—it is easier to keep the facts straight.

3. You should keep a notebook at home in which to jot down any questions or thoughts you might have, and take them to the doctor's office. The stress involved in going to appointments sometimes causes patients to forget their most important questions.

4. It is best to go to appointments with your spouse. Asking the questions is difficult enough. Remembering the answers is even more difficult. Two pairs of ears usually hear better than one pair. If your mate cannot attend, you can bring along a tape recorder.

5. It is essential for you to talk to your doctor about any concerns you have with him/her or with the staff. Infertility specialists are there to take care of their patients. If you do not feel cared for, then you are not getting the treatment you deserve. If your doctor reacts defensively or angrily to feedback, it is probably best to give that doctor one more chance. But if it happens again, you should probably consider changing doctors.

In a good working relationship between patient and physician, there is an abundance of mutual trust and respect. Both parties are hopeful about what they can achieve, but are realistic about the possibilities. In the pages that follow, we have included essays that address several different aspects of the doctor-patient relationship. Daniel Gottsegen, a well-respected infertility specialist, tells of the rewards and disappointments that he experiences in caring for his patients. He sadly acknowledges the fact that even the most dedicated physician cannot help all his patients conceive. Elizabeth Stanley, a former infertility patient who now coordinates an IVF program, tells what it meant to her to know that her doctor was really there for her. She identifies what he did that was most helpful to her and tells how she has attempted to incorporate his attitudes and manner in her own work. Patricia Pickett presents a less pleasant but equally real account of the doctor-patient relationship. Her essay reveals how some patients are forced to go from doctor to doctor, sometimes receiving both incorrect information and poor treatment.

On Becoming and Being an Infertility Specialist
Daniel Gottsegen

When I first entered medical school I had not decided what field I wanted to specialize in, but I knew which fields did not interest me. Among them were obstetrics and gynecology. However, by my third year of medical school, many fields that once seemed attractive no longer interested me. To my surprise, I found that I was drawn to the "happy" aspects of Ob-Gyn.

I began my fourth year of medical school with an elective in infertility. That four-week experience helping couples to conceive, convinced me that this was what I wanted to do. For me, no area of medicine could be more satisfying than helping couples become parents.

When I made the decision to specialize in infertility, I had no idea that the problem would touch me in my personal life as well. But soon after I began my residency, my wife and I decided that we were ready to begin a family of our own. Despite my awareness of infertility, we assumed that she would conceive promptly. After all, we were young and healthy, with no history of problems known to cause infertility. To our surprise and frustration, a pregnancy did not occur. Soon, I was in the ironic position of learning to be an infertility specialist and a patient at the same time.

For two years, Susan and I endured the frustrations and anguish of infertility. In retrospect, I realize that it was often easier for me to counsel and sympathize with my patients than it was to respond to my wife in the midst of this crisis. It was one thing to learn to perform an endometrial biopsy or a PK test, and another to watch my wife undergo painful or embarrassing procedures. Helping others conceive was exciting and gratifying, but those long, lonely mornings of awakening to our own temperature charts were exhausting and disappointing.

Our story has a happy ending. Amy and Adam, now fourteen and twelve, are the products of our efforts. I think that Susan and I have cherished them all the more because we tried so long to have them. Since then, when the going has been rough, we've been able to draw upon our years of struggle.

My professional life has also been enriched by infertility. While my practice is not limited exclusively to reproductive medicine, much of my work is in this field. Each day, I have the opportunity and the challenge of helping couples conceive. I celebrate with those who are successful and suffer with those whose best efforts (and my own) do not work out.

The recent and rapid advances in the field of infertility have made my work particularly exciting. This past year three colleagues and I started an IVF program, one which had a long and cautious gestation. I waited until I thought that our patients would have a reasonable chance of success and was pleased when all of the women in the first group had successful egg retrieval and fertilization. I was jubilant when one woman became pregnant!

Each positive pregnancy test—whether it be a result of minimal intervention or prolonged treatment—brings a big smile to my face. Still, I remain sobered by all the failures. For all the good news, there remain daily messages saying "Mrs. X called to say her period started—what next?" or "Mrs. Y (pregnant after four miscarriages) is now bleeding heavily."

With a busy practice, I worry that I am not always there for my patients when they need me most. I try hard to respond to them, particularly when they are most stressed, and to take the time to talk with them. We need to talk together about their feelings as well as about their treatment options. I have found time and again, that these talks help to lessen the frustrations.

And so, when I think back on my first year of medical school, I am relieved that I had an open mind. I feel fortunate to have found a specialty that is both professionally challenging and personally rewarding. My patients, and the very special work that we do together, enrich my life.

On Both Sides Now:
From Patient to Provider

Elizabeth Stanley

As I sit here watching my three children, I remember the pain and disappointment my husband and I experienced while trying to begin our family. After five years of trying on our own, we realized that it was time to consult a specialist. This was a very difficult decision for me because I was afraid of medical tests and felt uncomfortable with physicians.

Prior to being an infertility patient, my experience with physicians had been negative. Most were "stiff-collared" individuals who were difficult to talk with. I could not imagine speaking with them about such topics as intercourse and sexuality. Setting out to find an infertility specialist, I worried that I would find myself in the office of someone who would make me feel worse than I already did. And that was bad enough!

Despite my reservations, I finally got my courage up and started calling the offices of the recommended fertility specialists. I ended up making an appointment with the one who had the warmest and most helpful secretary. As it turned out, this was probably a very wise way to select my doctor since his secretary reflected a good deal about the way he ran his practice.

My first contact with Dr. G confirmed my sense that I had selected the right doctor. He was nothing like any of the doctors I had known or imagined. He greeted me with an apology for the long delay and soon after we met, shared with me the fact that he and his wife had had a personal experience with infertility several years earlier. I left his office feeling that we would work together in a warm, collaborative relationship.

The next year was filled with lab tests, post-coital tests and other measures of impaired fertility. I had a laparoscopy to determine whether or not I had any structural problems that could explain my infertility. Often I felt like I was on a roller coaster. Each time we thought that my problems had been corrected, another popped up. I was diagnosed as having ovulatory problems, a cervical factor, and a luteal phase defect. To make matters worse, my husband had problems as well.

My initial sense that I would be comfortable with Dr. G and feel that we were working together, was confirmed throughout my experience with him. It felt like a long, slow process, but he was always in there fighting—coming up with new plans for how we could overcome all of my problems.

The most difficult times for me were when I was on my own, having to wait. It was much easier for me to be active—to be making decisions or undertaking a new treatment plan. The waiting and wondering were so stressful. Again, I'm not sure I could have survived these times without Dr. G who always took the time to return my calls and to answer my questions, no matter how tedious and repetitive. Once he called to let me know that he had presented my case to a group of physicians and to tell me what they had to say. Another time, I had to leave his office because he was running behind and I had another commitment. That evening, he phoned me to apologize.

I can't emphasize how much Dr. G helped me to overcome my feelings of inadequacy. It was clear that he was very busy, but he always took the time for me. More important, he shared with me his feelings of frustration when we didn't succeed. At one point, he even suggested that I seek a second opinion, hoping he was missing something. I had no interest in doing this, feeling confident that no one else would have more to offer.

Having exhausted all other options, Dr. G and I decided it was time for me to try Pergonal. I did so and, initially, met with no more success than I had with the earlier, less dramatic treatments. Then, on my eighth Pergonal cycle, I decided to have a serum pregnancy test before my period was due. I felt that I could no longer stand the waiting and wondering, checking for blood every fifteen minutes, imagining that every time I blinked I felt a cramp. So, I had blood drawn, fully anticipating bad news.

I had often imagined how I would react to the news that I was pregnant. When it actually came that afternoon, my reaction was nothing like what I had anticipated. In place of the elation I had expected was disbelief. I had had so many disappointments that I could not believe my luck had changed. Surely, there had been a mistake.

There had not been a mistake. I was indeed pregnant. But for me, pregnancy after infertility proved to be difficult in many ways. First, there was the emotional stress of moving from being an infertility patient—with all the rights and privileges of that role—to being an ordinary OB patient. I felt that I needed more support than I was getting and feared that no one understood how worried and afraid I was.

As it turned out, my fears were well-founded. In my sixteenth week, it was discovered that I had an incompetent cervix and was already 75 percent effaced. I underwent a cervical cerclage and spent the remainder of my pregnancy fighting premature labor. Fortunately, I made it to thirty-seven weeks and delivered a healthy nine-pound baby boy.

As I mentioned at the start of this essay, I am now the mother of three, ever grateful that I found an excellent physician and that we were both persistent enough not to give up. I am particularly fortunate that our work together continued after the birth of my children. I am now the coordinator of the in vitro fertilization program that my physician directs. I have the opportunity to use what I learned from my experience as a patient in my work as a provider. I try to pay careful attention to the emotional needs of patients, remembering all too well the need to be informed, the need to have someone with whom to talk, the need to feel special.

I have found that patients are usually relieved that a coordinator is there to respond to them. Many times they will call to ask me questions that are important to them, but that they wouldn't think of taking to their physician. I keep a supply of greeting cards for different types of occasions and send them when circumstances warrant a compassionate gesture. I try to follow the progress of the patients and call to check on them from time to time. I make hospital visits when I can and enjoy meeting patients and holding their miracle babies when they are born.

As patient turned provider, I strive to be sensitive to the needs of couples after delivery. I know that they may feel disappointed when their relationship with their physician changes. While they may know and understand that their caregivers are now busy and involved with patients who are still trying to conceive, they still may feel rejected. For them, their physician has become part of the family—the third and very important member of the baby-making threesome. It is important to keep in mind, that though there is cause for celebration, there is also a loss involved.

I have heard a lot about the strained relationships that many infertility patients experience with their physicians and other caregivers. I suppose that given the stress inherent in all infertility treatment, some of this strain is inevitable. Nonetheless, I know—from both sides now—that the caregiver-patient relationship can be warm and gentle, laced with laughter as well as tears.

First, Do No Harm

Patricia Pickett

I first became pregnant during my junior year of high school and, having done so, subsequently married the father of my unborn child. Two babies and a great deal of physical and emotional abuse later, we divorced.

Sometime during the year following the birth of my second child, after my divorce, I noticed my periods becoming very erratic, sometimes lasting three days, more often, fifteen. Finally, during the Thanksgiving holiday, I was admitted to the hospital for an emergency D&C (dilation and curettage) to control what had become hemorrhagic bleeding. My doctor performed the procedure, assuring me that all went well and I was released from the hospital on the following day. The next month came without my menstrual cycle returning to normal, but I was unconcerned because the doctor had explained that it would probably take a few cycles for my periods to reestablish themselves.

After the third month passed without the appearance of a period, I did begin to worry, so I made another appointment with my doctor. He did a routine pelvic examination, found no abnormalities, and assured me that it was probably "just a little hormone imbalance." During our talk in his office, he also told me that he could prescribe hormones that would give me normal menstrual cycles, but that since I had previously had difficulty tolerating oral contraceptives, I might have the same type of problems with these hormones. He also said that my file indicated that I was unmarried, and that since I didn't wish to have a baby at this time, it seemed pointless to take the hormones. His whole attitude was "if it isn't broke, don't fix it." What I didn't realize was that something was "broke" and in need of repair.

About two years after my last visit with the doctor, the unexpected happened. I fell in love again and decided to get married. We discussed having children and were in agreement that we both very much wanted to have a family together. We knew that I might have difficulty conceiving, since I had not menstruated in over two years. Yet, at the time, nothing seemed insurmountable.

I went back to my doctor and informed him of my impending marriage, and of our desire to have children. His response was that I should have considered that when I refused the hormone therapy. I was shocked. He again examined me and found no physical abnormalities that he could detect, and advised me to go forth and multiply. That was it, no hormone assays, no basal temperature charts, no endometrial biopsies, no evaluation of any kind other than a pelvic examination. At this point I had become vaguely aware that I was no longer comfortable with, or capable of trusting, this doctor with my reproductive health. I searched for another physician.

My second doctor was very knowledgeable about obstetrics and gynecology, but not quite adequate in the field of reproductive endocrinology. His examination was much more thorough than the first doctor's, but still, no post-coital examination was performed, nor did he suggest a semen analysis for my husband to rule out combined factors. Months passed with still no pregnancy. Then, during a conversation with a physician friend, I asked if he knew of any local infertility specialists. He told me of another doctor who was affiliated with a local teaching hospital who treated only the most intractable cases of infertility, and only then on a referral basis. I discussed my problem with my friend, who then agreed to discuss my case with the other doctor.

A month passed and I forgot about that discussion until I received a letter bearing the letterhead of the local teaching hospital. I opened the letter and found what was, in essence, a summons to this doctor's office. I felt as though I had been granted an audience with the Pope.

Within minutes of my arrival at my third doctor's office, I was greeted and taken to the lab for extensive tests and analyses of my blood and urine. Then, I was taken to my new doctor's examination room. During the time that it took the lab to analyze the samples, this new doctor and I talked while he examined me. Within the course of three hours, he had the results of my tests and had easily diagnosed the problem. He explained what needed to be done and what options were open to my husband and me. Although my options were not limitless, they did include an exploratory laparoscopy and some very conservative surgery; monthly courses of Clomid; frequent blood tests or endometrial assays; or any combination thereof. We opted for the hormone therapy with the possibility of surgery later if necessary. Six months after my first visit with doctor number three, I became pregnant. Six days after we learned of my pregnancy, I spontaneously aborted a ten-week-old fetus.

At this time, doctor number three, whom I had come to view as our saviour, explained that he had accepted a more prestigious position with the hospital and was having to refer many of his patients to other doctors. He explained that his decision to refer me was due to the fact that I had proven that I could become pregnant relatively easily under the proper hormone regimen. Although I did not want to leave his care, I was glad that he had such an optimistic view of my problem. I made an appointment to see doctor number four.

On the first day of my appointment with doctor number four, we learned that he was tremendously overbooked. We waited for three hours, only to be told as I entered the examination room that the doctor to whom I had been referred was not in that day and that I would be seeing one of his associates. No one had told us of this arrangement and I was appalled that they would do such a thing without having first consulted me. I later found out that this "associate's" name was already on my chart! Needless to say, I was upset at having been shuffled to another doctor without anyone ever having asked my permission. Feeling our options were limited, however, I met with him. He swaggered into the examination room wearing a western shirt, belt buckle, and boots. He reminded me somewhat of our veterinarian.

Two months after our initial visit with doctor number four, I became pregnant again. We received the news on a Tuesday. The following Saturday I began to abort an eight-week-old fetus. We went to the hospital where I was immediately taken to the labor and delivery unit and unceremoniously deposited in a room located directly next to the delivery room. Doctor number four sauntered in looking as though he had just fallen off the hay wagon, with a demeanor that quickly told us we had disrupted his entire weekend routine. He snapped on his gloves, complained of a hole in one of them and muttered to the nurse, "She's aborting." Examination over, he left promptly without having spoken one word to my husband or me. The nurse helped me to dress and sent me home with instructions to return to the hospital if I began passing any tissue or bleeding more heavily.

We went home and I settled into our bed feeling drained both emotionally and physically. Seconds passed like hours, lying in that bed, still as death. I cried, questioned, and pleaded with God to let me have my baby. Several hours later we returned to the hospital where I fainted. We were taken directly back to the same little labor room, depressingly close to the delivery room. Some time later, we heard my doctor's voice in the hallway instructing a nurse to let one of the residents examine me because he had a delivery. Again, no one asked my consent to allow a stranger to examine me. The resident was as hurried and impersonal as my own doctor, and again I was sent home with nothing to numb the physical or emotional pain that I was feeling. I was told to be in my doctor's office early the following morning.

As instructed, we arrived early the next morning at my doctor's office, only to be told that it would not be open until one o'clock that afternoon. We left and returned in the middle of his obstetrics day. For two hours we waited in an office full of conspicuously pregnant women. I was not even able to lie down, nor to prop up my feet because there wasn t any room. My husband had to stand. When, finally, I was called to the inner office, I was examined and then given a pregnancy test because they weren't certain if I had aborted. I was then taken to the ultrasound room to see if a gestational sac could be detected. No one had mentioned the ultrasound. The doctor came in during the ultrasound, told me that I had definitely aborted, and then he left. No D&C was ever performed to determine if I had passed all of the products of conception, or to determine if there were any structural abnormalities that might have gone unnoticed in prior exams. I left his office and never returned.

About four months after my second spontaneous abortion, I began to have severe, incapacitating pain deep within my pelvis. Not knowing where to turn, I consulted our family physician (doctor number five). He examined me, went over my chart, and immediately referred me to yet another doctor for a surgical consultation.

Doctor number six also had a thriving practice, and I waited a long time before being called in to see him. During the examination, he noted that my left ovary was enlarged and tender with a palpable mass. Believing it to be of no consequence, he wrote me a prescription for Percodan, and suggested that I lose twenty pounds and pursue adoption. To make matters worse, he even asked if my two recent pregnancies had been the result of intercourse with my husband! He mumbled something about it being unusual that I had not become pregnant again. I left his office in tears, suffering from physical pain, and from humiliation. I could never have gone back to him, not after his treatment of me. Obviously he knew that I was in physical pain, hence the Percodan, but he compounded it with emotional pain and a crassness that I had never seen before in a doctor. Before going home, I went to my sister's house, to cry on her shoulder. She suggested that I see her gynecologist and, with much reluctance, I agreed.

My sister's doctor, doctor number seven, was a kind and competent man. But he, admittedly, had neither the training nor the experience in the field of infertility and endocrinology that doctor number eight had. Once again, I was referred to someone who, supposedly, could help.

We appeared at doctor number eight's office bright and early on a morning when I was in such pain that my husband planned to take me to the hospital if the doctor did not agree to see me. The receptionist told my husband that doctor number eight had taken that day off to tend to his wife, who was ill. My husband explained to her that his wife was also sick and needed to see someone, anyone. While he was explaining to the receptionist what was wrong, and what doctor number six had told me, a man standing in the waiting area, who seemed to be taking an interest in what my husband was saying, asked him where I was. My husband told him that I was in the car, and the man, who later turned out to be doctor number eight's associate, told him that he would examine me. He instructed his nurse to set up an examination room and then he came out to the car and took us both into his office.

This doctor did not know who we were, nor did he have my files. It seemed sufficient to him that I needed help. I was his first patient that day, and after he examined me, he spent time calling all my previous doctors' offices trying to obtain copies of my records, and explaining what he was doing. After he had gathered as much information as he could, he sent us to the hospital. The following day, he performed a laparoscopy on me and found that I had adhesions caused by either an acute pelvic infection that had gone untreated, or the last dying remnants of endometriosis. These adhesions had caused my left tube and ovary to become bound together and my uterus to become retroflexed. He also found indications of Asherman's syndrome, a condition sometimes caused by an improperly done D&C or induced abortion, which causes adhesions and scar tissue to form within the uterus. He said it was possibly caused by the D&C performed years previously by my first doctor. Using the laparoscope, he was able to remove many of the adhesions that had caused my uterus, left tube, and ovary to become distorted. He was also able to surgically tighten the ligatures supporting my uterus, thereby returning it to its normal position within the pelvis.

Ten weeks after the laparoscopy, I became pregnant again, this time, without the use of any hormones and without adhering to the treatment protocol advised by doctor number three. We received the news of my pregnancy on a Friday and two days later, I spontaneously aborted a six-week-old fetus.

It has been over two years since my last pregnancy. We have been in no hurry to board the fertility merry-go-round. Our long ordeal was so emotionally and physically draining that I am not certain that I have the courage to continue. Finally, however, we feel that we have a competent, and most important, a caring physician who helped us through a crisis and has stood by us since. This doctor has allowed us to have hope again, although it is still too frightening to be optimistic.

Although I will not pursue legal action against the doctors involved in the mistreatment of my condition, I firmly believe that the neglect I suffered both medically and emotionally, was criminal. More than one medical error was involved, and more than one busy physician had allowed an infection to proliferate within me. My fertility has been compromised, and perhaps even my life could have been in jeopardy if I had not gotten treatment. Though I firmly believe that no doctor ever intended to do me harm, I have suffered a great deal, and believe that much of it could have been avoided if only I had received proper treatment.

3
The Social and Emotional Effects of Infertility

INFERTILITY is a major life crisis. It puts enormous stress on the husband, the wife, and on their relationship. It is difficult, if not impossible, to escape its effects, since the fertile world is omnipresent, and doctor's appointments and treatment regimens consume so much of one's life. Couples in the midst of an infertility crisis think about little else. Their lives revolve around temperature charts, infertility specialists, medical procedures, and sex for procreation only. Even when couples go out together, in attempts to avoid the baby world, they frequently encounter a conspicuously expectant couple in a fancy restaurant, or a woman quietly nursing her newborn in the movie theatre.

From the time they are little girls, and become aware of pregnancy, women learn that their biological destiny is to bear children. In addition, although times are changing and men's and women's roles are now less rigid, women today have been socialized to anticipate raising their children—to be the primary caretaker. No matter to what extent a woman has developed a career or her professional identity, the image of herself as a mother is the psychological backdrop from which she operates. When a woman decides to have children and discovers she is infertile, her image of herself and, in many ways, her self-esteem, are shattered.

One's self-esteem is determined not only by external or societal reinforcements and cues, but also by internal cues that we perceive in our bodies. A healthy, well-functioning body enhances our self-image. Likewise, a physical problem or defect can contribute to a disturbed or negative self-image. The extent to which a man or woman's self-image is tied into his or her ability to produce babies, determines how much self-esteem will suffer as a result of infertility.

Women's bodies have a built-in calendar that is approximately twenty-eight days long. They may perceive bodily changes several times throughout the month, and these changes are intricately connected to their sexuality and to their physical comfort and well-being as well. When young girls complain about menstruation, they are often told by their mothers that the discomfort is worth it—that someday they will be able to have babies to hold and to love. They are paying a price for a future reward that will make it all worth while. When these girls grow up and become sexual, it is difficult, if not impossible, for them to separate their sexuality from their reproductive functioning. Whether women decide to have children when they are young, or to postpone childbearing, many approach conception as if it will come naturally and easily—the reward for which they have been waiting.

Infertility is usually a huge blow for a woman, particularly when much of her identity is tied into her ability to be a mother. Her sense of herself as a sexually desirable woman gets negatively distorted. She often suffers feelings of inadequacy, fearing that she is unlovable and unable to nurture. Women whose primary goal is to have children may become severely depressed. They begin to feel that their life is purposeless. They may experience themselves as unfeminine, damaged, defective. They tend to feel out of control and helpless. The longer infertility goes on, the more helpless they feel; and the more helpless they feel, the more depressed they become. Infertility is a vicious cycle.

A pervasive myth about infertility is that it is a woman's problem. In fact, one-third of all infertility is male related; one-third is female related; and another third is couple related. It seems sadly ironic that men who produce twenty million sperm at one ejaculation are only marginally fertile, and are considered to have an infertility problem. Twenty million sounds like such a large number, and, as everyone knows, it only takes one.

Men are not tuned into their bodies in the way women are. Physically, they feel the same, whether it is the first or the last day of the month. They have not been aware, nor have they been told countless times since puberty, that their bodies are preparing to make babies. Unlike most women, their identity is based primarily on their work and not on being a parent. Nevertheless, male infertility is extremely painful emotionally, and infertile men report over and over again the degree to which they feel defective as a man.

Fertility, masculinity, and potency are concepts that are often equated. It is understandable therefore, that when a man is given a diagnosis of infertility, his identity as a man suffers a real setback. He can easily feel impotent and emasculated. Sometimes men with no prior history of sexual inadequacy or dysfunction, become impotent for periods of time after they learn about their infertility problem. Even when it is the woman who is infertile, her partner can still feel his masculinity is threatened. Some men have the fantasy that if they were really potent, they would be able to impregnate their wives.

Infertility often challenges a couple's relationship. Couples who previously were warm, loving, and compatible, are dismayed to discover how much tension and distance has crept into their relationship since their diagnosis of infertility. And although infertility is a couple problem, the fact is that in two-thirds of the cases, the problem resides in one partner or the other. Often the infertile partner feels tremendous guilt, sometimes shame, about his or her condition, particularly if there has been a history of elective abortions, venereal disease, or drug or alcohol abuse. He or she is likely to fear rejection by the fertile spouse.

The fertile partner may also experience a range of emotions, including anger at the infertile spouse, alternating with guilt for having those feelings. Often sadness, anger, and fear become fused. In their worst moments, couples blame each other or suggest divorce, so that the fertile partner can remarry and make babies with someone else. Even when both spouses are infertile, there is a tremendous strain on the relationship. Each deals with the crisis and all its concomitant feelings in his or her own characteristic way.

Our society teaches women that it is okay to show their feelings, while men learn the opposite—that it is unmasculine to express sadness or vulnerability. Hence, a woman dealing with infertility typically expresses her feelings by talking frequently about her situation, crying, overtly worrying, and so on. Her spouse probably tries to be "strong" by not showing his feelings, and approaching the situation in a rational or logical way. Thus, men are often at a loss about how to help their wives in this crisis. They feel powerless, unable to comfort, and unable to change the situation.

Because they approach the crisis of infertility differently, husbands and wives often find it hard to communicate. Wives sometimes feel that their husbands don't understand how much they are suffering, and complain that they seem cold and indifferent. By contrast, husbands complain that their wives are too emotional. Couples begin to fear that infertility will destroy their relationship.

In reality, most marriages survive infertility and many grow from it. But in the midst of the crisis is much stress and strain. A couple's sexual relationship is probably the area that suffers the most. Because sex must occur on demand, rather than as a result of spontaneous feeling, it becomes a chore that is often dreaded. The notion of success (male orgasm) is substituted for the notion of pleasure. This can be particularly difficult for the husband since his self-esteem as a male has already been damaged by infertility. Maintaining an erection and reaching orgasm is not always possible, placing an even greater strain on the relationship.

Conclusive or absolute diagnosis of infertility are rare. And because there have been so many recent medical advances, doctors are reluctant to tell patients their situation is hopeless. Despite the wondrous results for many couples, other couples unfortunately find themselves in a prolonged crisis. They are unable to grieve the child they will not have, and so they cannot move on. Instead, life is put on hold and they may spend several years attempting to cope with the uncertainty.

In order to move on, couples must make decisions about when to stop treatment, and what alternatives they will pursue—either adoption or child-free living. They must grieve the loss of their fantasized child or children, despite the fact that some new treatment might just work, someday. Grieving can be a lengthy process for couples, one that in many ways began when they were first identified as infertile. It usually involves five stages, first identified by Dr. Elisabeth Kübler-Ross in her book *Death: The Final Stage of Growth:* denial, anger, bargaining, depression, and finally, acceptance. Couples move back and forth among the stages at various times during their crisis, not necessarily experiencing them in a linear fashion. Infertile couples can be helped in this process either by seeing a therapist (preferably together) or by being in an infertility support group.

The crisis of infertility does not vanish, even when a successful pregnancy is achieved. The emotions that it stirs up are too powerful to forget, and its impact is so intense that couples often wonder if the pleasure they feel in life and in each other will ever be restored. Most do find, however, that the pain diminishes over time, and that they are able to get on with their lives. Many discover, to their surprise, that infertility has brought some positive changes along with the hardship. Their relationship may be strengthened; they may feel more confident about their ability to cope with stress and loss; and they are likely to feel an enhanced appreciation of good health, good friends, and family.

While the decision to adopt or to live childfree helps a couple to move away from the crisis, neither of these resolutions cures infertility. What adoption cures, however, is childlessness. Childfree living offers other kinds of rewards. But neither option gives a couple the biological child that they set out to have. Sometimes, the fact that they have failed to accomplish a central life goal lives on with them. And while the process of having endured and accepted this loss may have been strengthening, they are still left with a lasting scar.

As clinicians, we try to help couples feel that they are not alone. Fertility is visible; infertility is not. Because infertile people are not obviously marked, they may be difficult to find and so they often feel alone and/or misunderstood. Though some people shy away from groups, we find support groups—couple or individual—the most direct and effective means of reducing isolation.

In working with couples, we try to help them see that, while they may react and express themselves differently, they are in the crisis together. Some need help setting time aside to discuss medical treatment and decisions about alternatives. Many couples need help expressing the sadness and anger that they feel about their predicament. This is especially important in situations in which one spouse has been diagnosed as infertile while the other is presumably fertile. We often attempt to help men feel more comfortable being with their wives when the latter are feeling particularly sad or depressed. We encourage them to just sit with their wives, to hold them, or to listen, without feeling that they must do something to take away the pain; their presence alone is healing.

Infertile couples are in the position of having to make a series of decisions: first about diagnosis, then about treatment, and later, for many, decisions regarding adoption, childfree living, or alternative reproductive procedures. Thus, an important component of counseling infertile couples has to do with decision making—helping them to make considered and informed decisions with which they can live.

As we will discuss in later chapters, infertility affects almost all relationships. We try to help infertile individuals and couples face difficulties as comfortably and effectively as they can, whether they be with physicians, family members, or friends. Relationships are important to infertile couples; otherwise they would not wish to be parents in the first place. The crisis of infertility often makes it clear to the people involved, just who is most important to them, and to whom they can turn for support and comfort. We try to help couples preserve their important connections with people and, occasionally, sever ties with those who lack understanding or empathy.

As mentioned earlier, infertility is a crisis in which identity and self-esteem are negatively affected. Early, unresolved family issues are often uncovered, sometimes regretfully. In short, individuals face conflicts and feelings about themselves that they did not anticipate. The extent to which they attempt to work out these issues—with or without a therapist—is purely a personal decision. But infertility does offer them the opportunity to get to know themselves a little better, and self-awareness can go a long way once the crisis has subsided.

Perhaps most important, we help couples say goodbye to a dream. Those couples who do not conceive need help mourning the loss of their biological children. We find that this loss often interfaces with other losses. Since infertile couples are often in their late thirties or early forties, they frequently face, or have faced, the illness or death of a parent. Infertility brings up both past and present losses, and each loss adds more poignancy and power to the others. Death, too, reminds us of our own mortality, which is our ultimate loss. Infertility forces us to face this painful realization.

Earlier in this chapter, we discussed the fact that women tend to have an easier time expressing feelings than do men. We are, however, surprised and delighted that most of the essays in this chapter are written by men. They offer a perspective that is not often viewed. Stephen S. Lottridge presents a poignant account of male infertility, while Emanuel Pariser takes a more philosophical look back on his infertility experience. Steven A. Adelman writes a candid account of what it feels like to be on the sidelines, speaking both as the fertile spouse and as a man, acknowledging that to some degree all men are bystanders to pregnancy and childbirth. Donna Ortenzi captures the disappointment of someone who had expected to have a family, and then encounters one road block after another to achieving that goal. And finally, Jane Clayton-Matthews addresses the impact of infertility on a marriage, noting ways in which a couple is strengthened as well as tested by the experience.

One Man's Infertility

Stephen S. Lottridge

I am an infertile man. I don't make babies. No doctor has ever said I *can't*; just that, well . . . adoption might be a nice idea. Or donor insemination—many couples are happy with that. Two of the more sanguine surgeons have clapped me on the back and said, "Go get 'em, tiger." But the fact is, that when I make love, babies don't get made.

My sperm, what there are of them, are immature, malformed, immotile. "Laid back," as a helpful reframer once said. Just "unready," as a cosmic thinker intoned. Still and all, whether unable or reluctant, my sperm do not do the one thing above all others that sperm are supposed to do: fertilize eggs.

They really do not seem like part of me, those sperm. How could they be? My father sired four children that I know of. My mother got pregnant the first month she ever tried. The problem, if there was one, was contraception, not fertility.

The biological connection in my family is powerful. I remember once, some eighteen years ago, sitting on a lawn swing with my brother, while our two sons—his by birth, mine by adoption—played on the grass. I looked at my arm lying on the back of the swing. Suddenly I realized I could not move it. It had no feeling. I felt a moment of panic, moving toward terror. Then, though I still could not feel it, the arm moved. As suddenly, I realized it was my brother's.

Many years later, I was walking down a city sidewalk. Unexpectedly, I saw my father walking toward me. I felt shock and joy—and then I realized it was a full-length mirror I was walking toward.

I and my father and brother are one flesh. But I cannot give that to any-one. My son will never see me in his body, or know himself in a brother's limb. The biological flow runs dry in me. Sometimes that knowledge aches and gnaws like an amputation. I long for my cut-off children.

I have known of my infertility for twenty years. It was the classic story for infertile couples. We tried for several months, a year, two, each month hop-ing, sure that it would work. And each month it didn't. Bewildered, fearful, we went for tests. At that time I didn't know, nor did anybody I talked to, that there were infertility specialists. I went to a urologist—the closest spe-cialist to the part of my body that might be in trouble. My wife went to a gynecologist, who found nothing amiss. I, however, turned out to have what was vaguely identified as "a low sperm count."

I vividly remember the indignity and pain of those appointments with the doctor. On my first visit I was asked—in a loud voice—to provide a sperm sample, and was pointed down the hall to the bathroom. The door didn't lock; it hooked. While I was trying manfully to "provide a sperm sample," I heard footsteps approaching the door, and then a loud voice shout, "Don't go in there; there's a guy jerking off in there." What sperm I had must have died on the spot, of shock and mortification.

That example is extreme. Most doctors and their staffs are much more sen-sitive to, and considerate of, the feelings of their patients. But that experience stands for me as a paradigm of the pain, exposure, helplessness, and shame that can attend infertility for men. The fact is that I felt, and can still feel these many years later, rageful, bitter, hurt, helpless, unfruitful, defeated, and sorrowful because I am infertile. And that experience also stands for me as a model of the incomprehension with which most of the fertile world responds to infertility and the emotional needs of infertile people.

At that time, like most men, I did not talk a lot about my feelings about infertility, nor did my wife and I discuss it much between ourselves. I went through an extended series of tests, which confirmed the original findings and also identified a varicocele. My (new) doctor discouraged me from having the varicocele operated on, however, and recommended that we try to adopt. In fairly short order, we applied to adopt an infant and, within a few months, by a lucky circumstance, became the adoptive parents of a baby son.

Our son thrived, and in many ways helped me forget my pain. But that pain remained, unresolved, until years later when, after many changes (including the end of my first marriage), I came to confront it again. In a new marriage, my wife and I faced our separate histories of infertility and our mutual struggle as an infertile couple.

Our lives were taken over by infertility. We lived in doctors' offices. We talked about infertility, worried about it, cried about it. No part of our lives was untouched by it. Our social lives were marked by it: we avoided gatherings where there were pregnant women or newborns; many times our depression and exhaustion held us at home; our conversation tended always toward the subject of infertility, and our views on abortion, birth control, and teen pregnancy were seen as cranky. Our relations with our families suffered: we were rarely cheerful; we talked always about the same thing; we could not explain satisfactorily why, in our late thirties and forties, we were *still* so bent on having children. And our relationship with each other was assaulted: the physical selves we had brought to each other in our meeting were violated by a multitude of invasive medical procedures; our sex life became metronomic; we fought, without point, out of our disappointment and irrational sense of betrayal. Each of us felt hurt, insufficiently tended, and profoundly betrayed by each other and by our own bodies.

I would like to say that through it all we maintained our good cheer and always stuck together, but we did not. Our anger and despair were often too deep and too ready. And our relationship was, after all, the locus of our pain. In classic fashion, I often wished my wife would respond less intensely just once in a while and felt that she overwhelmed me with her emotional chaos and demands. She, in turn, felt that I was uninvolved and aloof. What we were able to do was to realize, gradually, that nearly all our strife and unhappiness stemmed from our infertility. We began, then, to institution-alize our pain. We had what we called "The Friday Night Fights," in which we fought out our grievances and fears intentionally, so that they began to booby-trap us less.

One of the most important realizations we came to out of our struggles was that it is impossible to compare losses. It seems true, as much of the research suggests, that women who do not become successfully pregnant lose a more intimate and profound physical experience than do men who do not sire a child. There is also evidence to show that now, as in earlier times, women are more stigmatized for a failure to bear children than are men for not siring them. This does not mean, however, that a woman's desire to be a mother is larger or more intense than a man's to be a father. As with many other intense emotional events, men are trained to be less expressive—perhaps even less aware—of their feelings about being infertile, but that does not mean that they cannot or do not experience radical pain, loss, and dam-age to their vision of themselves.

I always thought I would sire children, out of my love, through my sperm. My love works; my sperm, it turns out, do not. In one of his books—*The 158 Pound Marriage*—John Irving's protagonist says he is a nat-ural at two things—wrestling and being a father. I never was much of a wrestler. But at being a father I thought I would be a natural. And I can be a father, but not "naturally." Infertility has become part of my identity and has altered it permanently. It is as if there were a label, appended to all the ways I might describe myself, to all the identities I might have, that says *infertile*.

I have struggled with the fear that if I am not creative reproductively, I cannot be creative in any way. If I cannot give my wife the baby she wants, I do not have anything worthy of giving to anyone I love. If I cannot continue the flow of generations, my existence on earth is fundamentally meaningless.

In unspoken ways, my family confirmed these feelings. They would not accept my infertility. I could feel their anger, especially that of my father. I think he felt it to be his failure, that he had sired a defective son, who could not carry on his line. But I also could feel, in his anger, his inexpressable compassion for me. I, in turn, felt anger at him for not having created me able to compete with him and join successfully the ranks of men.

Many years later, after his death, I came to understand that in some way my infertility had felt so debilitating for me because it seemed to confirm my worst male fear. What had made my ever-unsuccessful boyhood competi-tion with my father bearable was the image of myself, becoming a man, with a wife and family of my own. When I grew up, but could not sire children, it felt as if I were still not yet a man. Infertility counselors are at great pains to draw the distinction between fertility on the one hand and masculine vitality on the other. That distinction is crucial and true. I knew it in my head, and even felt myself to be strong and mature in many ways. But even so, because I was infertile I *felt* — as I suspect many men do at some level — that I was not a full-fledged member of the company of men, that I had still not left my father's shadow. It was only in seeing this clearly, after many years, that I was able to make my posthumous peace with him and to resolve those feelings of failure connected with my infertility.

And over our time together, my wife and I have come to a resolution of our infertility as a couple. We are the adoptive parents of a fine girl who thrives and finds our love. We no longer have, or need, our Friday night fights. But resolution and adoptive parenthood do not mean our infertility never happened — just that it does not loom so large in our lives now. We still hope, quietly, that my wife will get pregnant. We still comment on it, from time to time, or find each other pensive. I have an adopted son who is a fine young man. I have a baby daughter who is lovely as lovely can be. And yet, I am still an infertile man. I have resolved most of my feelings and I accept my infertility, but I will never, fully, be reconciled to it.

Reflections on Infertility: A Man's Perspective

Emanuel Pariser

I became a father after several years of infertility. My sons, now four and six, fill my life with pleasure and with challenges. As they move too quickly toward manhood, I think of the lessons that infertility taught me about myself and about other men. Those which stand out most have to do with lifelessness and denial of mortality.

When we were going through infertility treatment, I realized that I had always regarded myself as "outside of nature" or "over nature." I had rarely been bothered, except during brief illnesses, by my limitations as a "natural" being. I believed that my thoughts — clear and rational as they were — gave me control over my life. What I did not realize was that they rendered me lifeless.

Infertility made it impossible for me to remain lifeless. Suddenly, I felt angry, depressed, sad, powerless. I both pitied and blamed myself. I felt empty and oppressed. My conception of myself as competent and in control had been shaken to the core. I had lost my anchor.

But as I made my way through the experience, I began to wonder whether I might gain more than I'd lost. Infertility, cruel as it was, was teaching me that there was no shame in feeling. My feelings—good, bad, and indifferent—were my main moorings in the world. I realized that emotions could connect me to others and relieve me of the need to perform like a robot. I began to embrace my crisis and to feel that I could move on from it.

The second lesson that I learned from infertility has to do with mortality. When asked about their motivation for having children, many parents or parents-to-be, speak of the wish to carry on from one generation to another. I think that many people have a fantasy, tucked away in there, that their children will protect them from death. If they can live on in their children, they will not die.

Infertility hit me in the face with the reality of my own mortality. The threat that I might not father a child forced me to face the fact that "No matter how much you struggle and strive, you'll never get out of this world alive" (Hank Williams). Infertility felt like "the end of the line" and though that was frightening, it was liberating as well. Having looked death in the face, it was easier to live.

Which brings me to where I am now. Life with two boys is hectic and tiring. Quiet moments are few. Much of my time is spent refereeing or assisting. I am driver and audience and sportmate. A willing jack-of-all-trades.

What is most rewarding to me about being a father of two boys is that I have the opportunity to pass on to them the lessons that infertility has taught me. My sons will not grow up numb. They will not be obliged to act like robots. They will never be taught to keep emotions at arms' length.

I am raising men, not warriors.

Confessions of a Helpless Bystander

Steven A. Adelman

Somewhere in the middle of our six-year struggle to become a family I dreamt that I was inside my wife's womb. It was a spooky place: its luminous pink walls were decorated with gelatinous strands of dried blood and scar tissue. I remember feeling helpless and lost. There was nothing I could do and nowhere to go. A man imprisoned in a battered womb—to me this image captures my experience of infertility.

I've had a lot of time to think about making babies. The thoughts come first, then the feelings. It strikes me that the roles of men and women in reproduction are grossly unequal. The "male factor" necessary for pregnancy can be obtained, preserved, and transferred to a woman with relative ease. A man may give rise to a biological child with as little as a few minutes of involvement in the entire process. The woman is the integral partner in human reproduction—no child is ever born without the drastic transformations of a woman's body, mind, and life circumstances necessitated by pregnancy and childbirth.

Men stand on the sidelines while women are starting players in the game of human reproduction. Menstruation, missed periods, morning sickness, weight gain, vitamins, ultrasounds, amniocentesis, false labor, contractions and delivery—all these happen to women while their men look on. At best, a man plays a strong supporting role in the drama of his leading lady.

Thus, all couples, including fertile ones, experience "reproductive inequality." Each couple's individual situation shapes this imbalance in unique ways. My dream of imprisonment in a battered womb sums up my experience as a bystander in the process of reproduction.

It took us about eight months to get pregnant the first time. This pregnancy seemed out of control from the outset—no sooner was my wife pregnant than she began spotting. How could the development of my child be heralded by blood? The gynecologist reassured us that spotting was common in the early stages of pregnancy. Nonetheless, I felt terribly removed from what was happening in my wife's body, and I sought to overcome the feeling that I was losing control of the situation by consulting my medical school textbooks. I wondered whether the fetus was lodged somewhere outside the uterus—an ectopic pregnancy.

Reassured by my wife's physician that this was not the case, I made a short-lived peace with the notion that her pregnancy was out of my hands. In the tenth week we learned that my suspicions had been all too accurate: this pregnancy turned out to reside in her left Fallopian tube. When it ruptured we lost a lot: the fetus and the affected tube were removed, and the resulting scar tissue permanently impaired our ability to achieve another pregnancy by natural means.

This tragedy humbled me. My passionate desire to father a child seemed inconsequential. My attempt to use medical knowledge to avert a crisis had been casually thwarted with disastrous consequences. My wife had come close to losing her life, and it was unclear whether or not we would ever have a family of our own. This first pregnancy ruptured my illusion that working hard, planning carefully, and holding the proper values would enable me to realize all of my ambitions. I learned to take nothing for granted when it comes to bringing a child into the world.

For the next four years, I stood by my wife while she endured the physical and emotional hardships entailed by the diagnosis and treatment of our problem in conceiving a second pregnancy. Although this was my problem as well, it was her body, not mine, which had turned into a battle zone. At our behest, the forces of modern medicine declared war against an invisible resistance that doggedly prevented her eggs from passing into her uterus. It makes me sad to remember all of the insults and bodily intrusions: the biopsies, X rays, surgeries, and hormonal treatments. I tried to share as fully as I could the disappointment and heartache that each month's menses triggered in my wife. It was often difficult for me to fathom the depths of the pain she felt when her body refused to participate in one of its most basic functions: procreation.

Finally, we decided to pursue in vitro fertilization (IVF). The doctors told us we were ideal candidates for making a "test tube baby." The process was a grueling one: each cycle involved daily injections for a month, and multiple blood and urine tests, in addition to minor surgery, and a brief hospitalization we'd already undergone. In vitro fertilization renders some of the secrets of reproduction commonplace. Eggs are harvested, inseminated in a test tube, and the developing embryos are monitored and transferred into the uterus. The entire IVF process is carried out in a sterile hospital atmosphere of logic and scientific precision. Despite the veneer of order promised by technology, an undercurrent of intense and confusing emotions gripped us from the day of the first orientation meeting.

While my wife scurried back and forth to the hospital each day for testing and monitoring, I winced, knowing that the whole world was watching our private act. Secretaries called me with instructions about when and where to produce my semen. Aside from masturbating at the critical moment in a cramped bathroom in the hospital basement, my role in IVF was limited to injecting my wife with hormones at home and staying by her side in the brightly lit delivery room (how ironic!) while microscopic embryos were carefully introduced into her womb by the medical team. It was humiliating to feel that our ability to have a baby depended more on these masked professionals than it did on us.

Technology played a cruel trick on us. After one of the in vitro cycles my wife's pregnancy test was positive. We were ecstatic—multiple embryos had been transferred, perhaps she was carrying twins, or even triplets. The yoke of infertility began to lighten, only to grow heavier several weeks later when the tests began to indicate a problem with the pregnancy. Yes, lightning struck twice. The single developing embryo had moved upstream into her remaining Fallopian tube. Another ectopic pregnancy! Again, we lost the pregnancy and the tube, and all hope of an unassisted conception. It was as though we had treaded briefly on the soil of the Promised Land, only to be abruptly led away and banished for eternity. My wife felt betrayed by her body; I felt betrayed by God.

After several fruitless and disappointing years I began to consider adoption. While my wife's body and spirit were exhausted and ravaged by the infertility war, I mustered up enough energy and interest to explore the alternatives and set the process in motion. At first, I feared that adoption would be as elusive as a successful pregnancy. Another failure would be devastating.

Happily, I was wrong. The decision to adopt liberated me. The process provided a wonderful opportunity for me to be personally active and involved in the creation of our family. Ineffective as a sire of children, I felt mended and restored by my efforts to amass all the necessary medical, legal, and personal documents. Less than a year after we started the adoption process in earnest, our infant son arrived.

Sometimes I feel so excited about being the father of a baby boy that I imagine what it would have been like if he had grown inside of me. Although I will never forget the womb-prison of my dream, I don't feel as though I am living there anymore.

The Goal I Cannot Dis-own

Donna Ortenzi

I have felt since I was quite young, that I never had a true sense of "family." My parents had a very stormy marriage that lasted until I was eighteen years old. I am the middle child with a brother on each end. We all suffered as a result of our parents' problems, but my brothers had each other and didn't care much about me. Somehow, I managed to survive.

When I married at age twenty-nine, I thought, "Here at last, is the beginning of my family." My husband, Al, had two sons from a previous marriage. So in some ways, I had an instant family. I worked out a nice relationship with the boys and enjoyed the time I spent with them. But from the start, Al and I were clear that we wanted to have a child together.

We knew of one obstacle to pregnancy: Al's vasectomy. Soon after we were married, he underwent surgery in an attempt to reverse it. Initially we believed that the surgery had been successful, but as it turned out, Al had to have a repeat procedure one year later. Things went better this time and soon after the surgery, Al had a sperm count that was in the low normal range.

Because we were focusing on Al's problem and assumed that I was fertile, I did not see an infertility specialist. Nonetheless, my doctor did begin a basic work-up and started me on fertility drugs. Three years passed with no success. My doctor kept blaming my husband's low sperm count, but had me continue with tests and medication.

Our frustrations grew. Sex became a chore rather than a pleasure. Our marriage suffered and we sought professional counseling. Soon we were back on track sexually, but I was in a good deal of pain over this whole issue. I now had all sorts of reasons why I could not conceive. Often I thought I was being punished for something I did wrong. Other times I wondered if God was trying to tell me I'd be a lousy mother. Alternatively, I wondered if this was my protection from giving birth to a seriously ill or deformed child. Out of hope and out of steam, I decided not to pursue the matter any longer. I felt that I had best accept my fate and resign myself to the fact that I would never be a mother.

My therapist is a wise man and he challenged my decision to give up. I had to admit to myself, as well as to him, that I still longed for a baby. He suggested that the time had long since come for us to see an infertility specialist.

Al and I began seeing a reproductive endocrinologist four months ago. From the start he has been compassionate and responsive. He acknowledges that we have been through a great deal, but encourages us to continue treatments. He is hopeful that husband insemination will work and we are ready to give it a try. I am working hard to maintain some hope in the face of great despair.

This roller coaster ride called infertility has caused me to question myself and my basic assumptions about the world. Often I have tried to convince myself that family doesn't matter. That I can be fulfilled as a stepmother. Again, I've looked at it fatalistically and declared it was meant to be.

But in my heart of hearts I want to be a mother. I am exhausted, but still I long to hold a little one. To watch him learn to walk. To help her with her homework. To be the driver and the toy picker-upper and the tooth fairy. Because my goal is clear, because it is of great value to me, I cannot dis-own it.

And so I persist, summoning up the energy to try again. And then again.

Infertility: One Couple's Experience

Jane Clayton-Matthews

My husband and I recently celebrated our second wedding anniversary and five years of being "together." However, it has occurred to me that the whole notion of being together takes on new meaning when a couple is dealing with infertility.

First there is denial. When is it that a couple decides that something is "wrong"? In our case, I was already beginning to grieve the loss of mother-hood while my husband continued to joyfully anticipate the coming of a pregnancy in any given month. This made it very difficult to share the problem in the way that we do today.

As each monthly cycle ended with the dreaded menstrual period, I began to feel more and more hopeless. After a year of riding the cyclical roller coaster and the associated feelings of failure and inadequacy, I realized that I was depressed. Compounding the difficulty was the fact that I had put my career plans on hold and was in a perpetual state of suspended animation. As for my husband, he had recently completed his Ph.D. which involved a ten-year effort, and was beginning a new job intended to develop him profes-sionally. I was longing for a job I had not expected to wait for—mother-hood. At the same time, I was postponing important career decisions while my husband was pursuing his own.

The decision to begin an infertility work-up evolved out of my sense of fear and hopelessness. This seemed to convince my husband that something was "wrong." At the same time we became aware that tension, distance, and discomfort had developed between us. Until our infertility problem emerged, we had enjoyed a level of intimacy that allowed for spontaneity, laughter, and a relaxed lifestyle. Now our days were numbered by the calen-dar, temperature charts, ovulation predictor kits, and medical procedures. It became so difficult to talk with each other without discussing my infertility that we began to lose all of the aspects of our relationship that brought us together in the first place. Our sexual relationship changed from a pleasure-seeking activity to a tension-producing event that was mechanical and planned. This was a frightening realization and the possibility that it could be endless was overwhelming.

We came to believe over time that it might be helpful to see a therapist. Couples counseling had been useful in the past and since I have a background in psychology, it was easier for me to understand the pressing need to regain a sense of control over our lives.

What we learned through counseling is that couples go through stages when they are dealing with infertility, and these stages are not necessarily entered into simultaneously by the couple. Just as I was shouldering the burden of hopelessness for both of us, my husband was feeling pressured to be the "hopeful" partner. What needed to happen was for my husband to allow himself to grieve and for me to be able to feel hope and not give up on the situation. Otherwise, our infertility would continue to polarize us and we would drift further apart. We discovered that although we both felt periods of grief alternating with periods of hope, we had become trapped in our respective roles. When we could each allow ourselves to experience both sets of feelings we readily grew closer to each other.

I remember feeling surprised but so loving toward my husband when he returned from a business trip one evening and acknowledged feeling sad about seeing a child on the plane ride home. I found myself telling him not to worry, that I would eventually become pregnant. Here I was communicating hope for the first time! It became clear that evening that we had taken over parts of each other's feelings.

My husband and I have never been closer than we are now. The infertility work-up is a grueling, difficult process and we are right in the middle of it. The "problem" lies with me and not my husband. I am gradually learning how to cope with my feelings of inadequacy. I am also trying to make peace with what we are going through and the fact that I cannot control the outcome. I am not a very patient person and I like to be in charge of my life. I am also a goal-oriented person who chooses to make plans for the future. These character traits are in direct conflict with the waiting one must endure when dealing with infertility. Consequently, this may be the greatest challenge I face in my life. I can't help but "wait" each month in the hope of achieving a pregnancy. However, I am pursuing career interests and not placing this vital part of my life on hold.

As for my husband and me, a great deal has changed for us despite the fact that we do not have the prospect of a child in front of us as we had hoped. The difference now is that *we* are going through this process even though it is my body that is producing the difficulty. My husband has been with me through a painful D&C and endometrial biopsy, and will be with me when I have a hysterosalpingogram next month. My pain is his pain and his presence gives me the courage to press on.

I am firmly convinced that this difficult ordeal has strengthened us as a couple. As we celebrated our second anniversary I wondered what life would have been like had it been "easy" for us, and had I become pregnant right away as we had planned. Certainly we would have gained a child, but we also would have missed the opportunity to experience the deeper reserves of our love, strength, and commitment to each other.

4
Relationships with Family and Friends

O NE of the biggest challenges facing an infertile couple is relating to family and friends. Unlike other personal problems that can more easily remain private, infertility plays some part in most interpersonal relationships. Friends and relatives become pregnant; parents ask when they are going to become grandparents; strangers ask innocently if a couple has children. And invitations to baby showers arrive with regularity.

Infertile couples must make a decision, very often an evolving one, regarding how public they will be about their infertility. Some feel that it is a very private matter to be shared with only a few close friends or family members, if anyone. Others feel much more comfortable letting people know about their infertility, believing that secrecy only causes additional stress.

Regardless of how public or private they decide to be with their infertility, couples find that this issue is more complicated than they anticipated. Those who choose privacy frequently find they are troubled by all the lies that they have to tell—lies about where they are going when they have to rush off for doctor's appointments; lies about how they are spending their money or about what they are saving it for; and most painful of all, lies about their interest in having children. It is certainly difficult to act casual or indifferent about something that is the focus of nearly all their emotional and physical energy.

Couples often have differences regarding the privacy issue. They have to negotiate who and what to tell. Sometimes it is the husband, sometimes the wife, who demands more privacy. Particularly stressful is the situation in which one member of a couple insists upon total secrecy when the spouse wants to be more open. This comes up most often in cases of male infertility; men tend to feel more shame about their problem and to ask or expect their wives to camouflage it. In particular, couples who are considering donor insemination usually choose to keep it a relatively private matter, telling only very close friends and immediate family members, if anyone at all.

Couples who decide to be more public about their infertility generally feel less burdened. They do not have to live with a giant secret that overshadows all their interactions. Nonetheless, they do find that being open about their problem can be troublesome. They must constantly consider how much they wish to discuss their infertility and with whom. Being open does not mean they decide to tell everyone. And telling people that they have a problem does not mean they must discuss all the details.

Infertile couples, whether public or private about their infertility, must deal with the constant series of pregnancies that surround them. Being in their childbearing years, by definition, means that friends, siblings, colleagues, and neighbors are likely to be having babies. The infertile couple struggles between not wanting to further isolate themselves by attempting to avoid pregnant people and infants, and not wanting to intensify their own suffering by knowingly placing themselves in painful situations. Sometimes couples, in hopes of escaping the baby world, attend adult functions, such as cocktail parties, only to find that a couple who gave birth the previous week shows up with their newborn. Though it is possible to avoid the baby world on many occasions, sometimes even the most carefully considered situations prove to be more upsetting than expected.

There are certain experiences that are especially difficult for infertile couples, some of which can be avoided and some of which cannot. They include:

The News. Learning that a friend or family member is pregnant is always emotionally difficult. Some infertile couples feel that it is easier to be with a full-bellied woman than it is to learn that someone is pregnant. Yet although the news is always painful, certain factors make it more or less so. Infertile people generally prefer hearing about a pregnancy from the woman herself, rather than learning the news through the grapevine. If she also acknowledges their pain, in the telling, it helps. When the pregnant woman has had a history of infertility or pregnancy loss, the news is more bearable, sometimes even welcomed.

The Pregnancy of a Sibling. The pregnancy of a sibling, particularly a younger sister, is exceptionally difficult for most people experiencing infertility. It is even worse when this pregnancy heralds the arrival of a first grandchild. There is a sense that the natural order of things has been violated. The infertile sibling feels isolated from his or her family, unable to celebrate or participate in an important family milestone. Even when family members know about the infertility problem, they are often at a loss about how to deal with the infertile couple. Family ties are important. So are the feelings of all people involved. It is a difficult task for relatives to temper their excitement about the impending birth, with their concern for the couple in distress about their infertility.

Infertile couples experience a difficult dilemma, particularly around holiday time or important family events, such as anniversary parties. The infertile couple is caught in an emotional bind. They already feel isolated from most of the world. They want to be with their families, yet their pain is even greater when they are among pregnant siblings, or with very young nieces and nephews.

The Baby Shower. Every infertile woman comes to live in dread of invitations to baby showers. While it becomes nearly impossible to sit among women who are happily speaking about pregnancy and babies, it is also upsetting to keep declining invitations. Infertile women fear that their inability to attend showers means that they are selfish people, unable to give. They fear also, that by not attending baby showers they will further isolate themselves from others and permanently damage important relationships.

Most infertile women discover, however, that they can skip baby showers and still have friends. Some find that they simply need to stay away from pregnant friends and relatives for a time, and that those who care about them will understand. Others feel that the relationships are too important to be lost to infertility. Their solution often is to spend time alone with the pregnant friend, rather than be part of a large celebration.

In fact, friendships are sometimes lost over infertility. Depending on the degree of insensitivity, and a couple's willingness to tolerate it, the friendship may or may not endure. In these instances infertile couples, and most often the woman, decide that the relationship is not worth the discomfort they experience when they are together. When fertile friends do their best to socialize without their babies, to talk primarily about "adult" issues and be sensitive to their pain, the infertile couple is usually more eager to preserve the relationship. Similarly, relationships with family members may or may not endure depending on the sensitivity of the relatives. But because it is easier to leave friends than to leave family, family relationships are more likely than friendships to survive infertility.

Infertile couples not only face the challenge of dealing with other people's pregnancies, but they must also field questions, comments, and advice about their childless situation. Those who don't know about their infertility ask the couple when they are going to have a baby. Or they make crass remarks, probably not intending to hurt, suggesting that their lifestyle is self-centered. Having children is one personal area of people's lives that is frequently treated like public business.

When others know about a couple's infertility, they may offer an assortment of comments and questions that can be difficult to handle. Well-intentioned family members and friends offer advice. Someone always knows someone somewhere who has a miraculous cure to offer. Or they ask questions, wanting to know the latest details of a couple's treatment.

It can help infertile couples to keep in mind that the subject of their infertility is not only difficult for themselves, but also for those close to them. Family members, in particular, often find themselves in a no-win situation. If they ask too many questions or give unsolicited advice, they run the risk of seeming intrusive. If they say little, then they can be accused of disinterest, of avoiding the subject, or even worse, of diminishing the importance of the problem. It helps when infertile couples can give clear cues to family and friends as to what they want to talk about and with whom. As their treatment becomes more or less stressful, as their prognosis becomes more or less hopeful, they may experience a shift in their need to talk with others.

In addition to the toll it takes on them personally, infertile couples recognize that their infertility also has an impact on those most dear to them. They know that infertility alters the intended make-up of their extended families, and all involved experience feelings of loss. As parents age or become ill, the unalterable fact of the couple's infertility becomes even more painful.

In spite of all the stress that may accompany relationships with family and friends, couples find that infertility usually is not destructive. Relationships that matter tend to survive, and many are actually enriched by the experience. Infertile couples may find that they can talk more openly and honestly with family and friends about a range of subjects once they have made their way through infertility together. And while there are often some hurtful and insensitive remarks to endure, couples are also touched by the support and caring that loved ones can offer.

Relationships born of infertility often become the silver lining in the dark cloud. When infertile couples form friendships, initially based on their shared experience, the pain is diminished. Though some of these relationships are short-lived, many do survive and flourish. As infertile couples go on to become parents, whether it be by birth or adoption, it is special to share that experience with others who have traveled down the same road, and who can truly share their joy.

We include in this chapter three essays that address different aspects of the infertile couple's experience with family and friends. Kathleen Weaver has written two pieces: "Mother-in-Love" describes feelings of closeness toward her mother-in-law, and the pain she feels about not being able to provide her with a grandchild; "Covenant of Tears" illustrates the hostility, rarely written about but often felt, that infertile people can feel toward their fertile friends. Finally, in "Can Anyone Understand?", Louise Fulton captures the pain, loneliness, and longing she feels, particularly around young children and pregnant women.

Mother-in-Love

Kathleen Weaver

In-laws, particularly mother-in-laws, are the subject of jokes, nasty discourses, and even marital problems, but rarely praise. On my wedding day I trembled—not over possible marital problems of the wedding night—but over pleasing my future in-laws whom I had come to love. I could never have foreseen, even on that most joyous day of my life, the wonderful relationship that would ensue. Nor could I have imagined the tragedy that we would face together.

My in-laws watched me grow up through high school and college wondering if I would be their eldest son's wife. When the happy day came it was a difficult transition for them. It meant giving up George, their firstborn, the one for whom they had waited after three years and two miscarriages, wondering, as we do now, if they would ever be parents.

There were many happy times in our first two years of marriage. I remember my in-laws' first visit to our home in Florida. Before they arrived, I cleaned and cooked for two weeks straight. The baseboards and light-switches would never again be as spotless. I spent hours baking old fashioned cheesecake—one of my father-in-law's favorites. They raved about our apartment and the meals and we spent the days sightseeing and making memories. On a trip north, we traveled with Mom and Dad to a beautiful mountainous area upstate. Falling snow hushed everything save our laughter, as Mom insisted on wrapping her scarf around my head to keep me from catching cold.

These were precious times. But so were the sad ones: the time we flew home for Grandmother's funeral. Dad, not usually expressive, hugged George with tears in his eyes. And when my mother died, Mom brought me a beautiful vase of flowers, set it on the table, and held me as if I were her child.

As months and years went by, these experiences drew us closer. Soon Mom referred to me not as her "daughter-in-law" but her "daughter-in-love." After my mother's death, I would forget at times to say mother-in-law to people, referring to her as my "mother."

When George and I first discovered we had an infertility problem we were reluctant to tell his parents, fearing we'd disappoint them. But as time went on, we realized that it would be far more damaging not to tell them. Once we involved them, they responded as parents whose children needed them, never acknowledging their need to be grandparents.

Mom and Dad were there for us during the hardest times. When I had two surgeries during a three-month period, Mom held my hand in the emergency room, nursed me back to health, and allowed me to express my feelings when the struggle felt like too much to bear. Dad visited me in the hospital, often coming straight from work after an hour's drive.

Our struggle continues and so does our warm and loving relationship with George's parents. In fact, it has grown. Now when they come to our home to visit, I don't feel the need to be perfect. If there is dust on the lamp or a fingerprint on the light switch, I know they are there to visit us and not to inspect. Sometimes I will even buy the cheesecake. I know how sincere and unquestioning they are.

Even with their tremendous love and acceptance, at times I feel I could not have failed my in-laws more. How can I look into eyes that adore my husband and tell them his special talents might die when he dies? Of their children, my husband resembles his father the most closely, not only in looks, but in personality. How can I tell my dear father-in-law, one of the kindest, most intelligent men I know, that these traits may not be passed on? They endured childlessness and miscarriage early in their own marriage. How can I sentence them to this pain once again? How can I make them barren grandparents? And how will we feel, as their joy explodes when George's siblings give them the grandchildren we so desperately want to give them.

George says that if we adopt they will love our child because it will become a part of us—as he learns to play the piano and excel in math like George; as she develops my sensitivity and language skills.

I sit wondering at times if it wouldn't be easier to have wretched in-laws—to hate them and feel no remorse over disappointing them. Other times I marvel at the cruelty of this disease that plagues generations, not just individuals. And sometimes I just dream . . . of placing into my father-in-law's arms the next generation.

Covenant of Tears

Kathleen Weaver

I have felt the stabbing jealousy hundreds of times. It sears my soul until love burns away and hatred fills its empty space. I feel it when the announcement is first made with fuss and elation. And I feel it for months after the event.

Though the faces change, the scenario remains constant. Their bulging stomachs surround me as I smile and nod agreeably, all the while wishing them ill. In my sadistic mind, I heap misfortune on them, cursing them with my pain—pain no one should suffer. Prudence snaps me back to a guilty reality. What monster have I become?

Conquering it seems hopeless. The more kindness I show, the hotter it burns. Outwardly I pour love, inwardly hate rages. I ask myself how, when no one has wronged me, do I find such wretchedness within me. This disease controls my very being—body, mind, and soul—and I am prisoner to its bitter lot.

My freedom began today—with a friend who made the same announcement. She spoke not in the usual attention-getting fashion of broad grins and little empathy. For on one of her happiest days, she told me the news with tears in her eyes—tears for me—and with a prayer in her heart, committed in my struggle.

Sympathy had not borne these tears, but a covenant of love and hope. And suddenly, the love and joy I never envisioned feeling, welled up in my heart and soul, leaving no room for hate. That which I'd feared lost was awakened by someone who felt my pain, though not having experienced it. Inside I felt *her* happiness as my own and it gave birth to a spark of hope—for the future of my soul and body.

Can Anyone Understand?

Louise Fulton

It all seems so hard to explain. Yet it couldn't be more important to me. Take last weekend, for instance.

Just what I need, I thought. An adorable little three-year-old boy. Perky, bright, curious, aware of his appeal. Little Tommy came over with his parents, Marcia and Harold, when Harold stopped by to see my husband, Alex. I hadn't met any of them before.

"Where's the little girl?" Tommy asked.

"I think you have the wrong house," his mother said, amused. Marcia was cheerfully pregnant, eight months pregnant, she explained, with child number two. She was wearing a pink-pearl-studded knit top, gathered to emphasize her fullness.

Little Tommy turned to me, surprised. "Why *don't* you have a little girl?" he asked.

"I don't know," I said with a wry grin. I was surprised at my comfort; I'd answered Tommy's blunt question with the simple truth. For more than three years, we'd been trying to have a baby and we still didn't know why we couldn't do it.

"Not everyone wants to have children," interjected his mother. I felt less comfortable about that one and didn't say a word.

Tommy coped with the disappointment about the little girl. He played with Michael the Bear and later, when my husband suggested it, with our two little pink stuffed pigs. Alex had given me the twin pigs—one with a blue ribbon and the other with a pink ribbon—when I started the fertility drug Clomid. The gift was a little celebration joke, since Clomid increases the chance of multiple births.

But now I felt awkward and exposed. How do I explain why we have all these stuffed animals, I thought, not to mention the obvious twins, the boy and the girl pig. I wondered if I was being oversensitive. Yet recently, when a celebrity announced she was having twins, my first thought was "Clomid." Why yes, I had mused, she must have needed fertility drugs. No privacy here.

Now I sat down and talked with the mother, with Marcia—a full-time social scientist at a major university. She was coping just fine with her teaching, research, motherhood, pregnancy, and whatever else. If I had given up motherhood for a career, well, I didn't have to.

"I used to work twelve-hour days," she explained. "But now I can only work eight-hour days." She had put Tommy in a day care program from an early age. I guess that helped.

Later, Tommy asked me again: "Why *don't* you have a little girl?" My goodness, Tommy, stop, you're breaking my heart. There's nothing I'd rather do right now than bring out our little girl to meet you.

"We do have a little girl *doll*," I offered. But Tommy wasn't interested.

Marcia volunteered another explanation: "They have a lot of computers." Now what do you reply to that?

Actually it was ironic, since I'd used that one some years before. An acquaintance had asked about kids, and I'd joked that "We are having computers instead—last week there was only one, and now there are two."

This week we could have seven-hundred computers and it wouldn't help.

Later, Tommy left with his parents, jumping, running, and hopping down our front steps. I watched them get in the car. Mother settled herself carefully, aware of Tommy's almost-born brother or sister. Maybe Tommy would be the one to "have a little girl."

Goodbye, Tommy.

*

It seemed like a little twig, barely clinging by a single root to the side of a steep, bare, windy cliff, winding into a crack in the sheer rock wall. That was the pregnancy I finally had. There was really no hope for it; it was going to miscarry, to die.

In silent grief, I listened to it; the pregnancy hormone signal got weaker and weaker. It was a peep, a squeak, a feeble cry, a plea for help from our tiny and doomed little person.

How can anyone stand this? I wondered. The child will vanish, our longed-for child; it's there right now, it exists, it's alive, but it's getting feebler, it's fading out—first a shout, now a word, now a whisper, and now, nothing.

*

Can anyone but an infertile person know what it's like?

The worst part is the uncertainty, not knowing if you will *ever* see that child you want so badly. You see the future stretching out before you, a total blank, an unknown quantity. Maybe it will happen—dare you hope?—and quite possibly it will not.

Another sensation may accompany the blankness. Its color is the bleakest gray and there's a dull hiss in the background, like white noise, harsh and meaningless, but more muted. A feeling starts in the stomach as a kind of heaviness and moves up, leading to a tenseness in the shoulders and a constriction in the throat.

If we had a child, would I ever forget that feeling? Perhaps it's too strong and too painful to ever be remembered completely. In the same way, the memory of physical pain may leave only a trace of its horrible power—the power that, at the time, made you vow to do anything, anything at all, to make the pain go away.

I had a dream last night; I stole someone's baby—sort of. I wasn't sure what it meant. But it was nice to have the baby.

I was at the college and was watching after the little infant, a tiny thing bundled in white, while the mother went somewhere on the other side of the grounds. The baby and I were outdoors under the full late-summer trees, surrounded by scattered sunshine. I decided to drive the mother's car over and meet her near the administration building.

Hugging the baby to me, I climbed in the long old sedan and then settled the baby on the passenger seat. We drove a little way. Then something went wrong with the car, so I put the baby safely on the ground under a tree. I began wrestling with the car which was now writhing like a large animal, out of control.

I realized that the car wouldn't work and that the mother no longer knew where we were. I hugged the baby to my side and decided to keep the baby—at least for a little while.

*

The ovaries to the woman: "You want us to go through this whole thing again? We worked so hard last month and, after all that, nothing."

Reply: "It's just as hard for me. Tonight I was at the mall, near the 'Stork Time' shop where I got Alex the 'Father to Bee' T-Shirt, you know, the silly one with the buzzing bee on the front. The last time I was near that store, I was pregnant, happy, hopeful, a wonderful time. Our baby was there at last, growing, alive, a miracle.

They put the T-shirt in a box and I drew a picture of me and Alex and the baby on the cover with part of the message going: YAAAAY! Tonight, I just got sullen as we walked past the store with some friends. Our baby is gone. God, it's depressing."

"So here you are," the ovaries say, "Doing the urine test again for the ovulation signal. Lovingly, carefully, we'll admit that. But all of this is so much work for you, for us too. Is it really worth all this grief?"

"I don't know," the woman replied grimly. "All I can do is keep trying. It's so hard, but I force myself. I'm a mother fighting for the life of my child. What else can I possibly do?"

*

Now, I imagine, I'm sitting here, sitting in my future on the other side of the menopausal fence, old and childless, creaky and bent, an ancient tree above me, withered and drooping. The sadness returns, it's here once again, and again and again. It will never end; I'll be sad all my life.

Now I think it through for the thousandth time, what we did at the end of the 1980s, the last chance we had, the one that we blew. I run through it over and over again: what we didn't see, what we didn't do, what we did do but did too late. We certainly tried—I'm glad of that. But we didn't know enough back then; no one did.

Still, it doesn't stop the regrets.

The life that wasn't, the rainbow of possibilities, the happiness lost, the squeals of joy, the runs through the woods, the picnics by the beach, the homework at night, the learning, the games, the tiffs and squabbles, the joyous growth from grief and tears, the discoveries of life and of self. These are the memories that never were, played over and over and in living color, under the creaking tree in the grayish aging mind.

But it's not over yet. I read it once again: "Three out of five infertile couples will eventually have a baby." There's hope for us, I tell myself; the odds are actually in our favor. Well, maybe a bit lower—we're older than most—but there's definitely a chance. I smile as I picture our success: our little infant, cooing and kicking happily. Yes, we've got to keep trying. Whatever it takes. And maybe, oh maybe, we'll be among the lucky ones.

5

Infertility and Career

IN choosing a career, most people give some thought to how and when children will (or will not) fit into their work lives. First, there are important considerations regarding timing. Some couples elect to pursue a family first, believing that a career should wait; others prefer to be comfortably settled in their work before embarking upon the full-time job of raising a family. Couples look, also, at how a particular career fits in with childrearing. Does it allow for part-time work? Flexible hours? Can work be done at home? For men, the issue of time commitment may be important, but is secondary to financial considerations. Most couples want to know that their primary career can generate enough income to support a family.

When a couple encounters infertility, earlier career decisions are called into question. Women who passed up the opportunity to go to graduate school may feel doubly cheated, lacking a baby as well as a satisfying career. They may wonder if an interesting job, or school, would somehow lessen the sting of infertility. Career women often look back with regret and self-blame, fearful that they have passed up their only opportunity to have what really matters. Men who worked hard to attain positions that would comfortably support a family, may question what their efforts were all about.

In addition to questioning earlier career decisions, infertility interferes with current job performance, and with plans for job change or advancement. Frequent, and precisely timed, doctor's appointments cut into even the most flexible work schedules. Work related travel becomes difficult if not impossible.

The emotional stress of infertility diminishes the energy that many people have for their work. Even those who are generally enthusiastic feel depleted by the tests and procedures, the questions, and the uncertainty involved. In addition, relationships with pregnant colleagues and clients are understandably strained.

Individuals considering a job change or advancement also find that their decision is affected by their infertility. It is difficult to begin a new job in the midst of a treatment, because of the time involved in new work settings. Women may feel they are being deceitful taking a new job while involved in treatment, since pregnancy, their most immediate goal, would surely complicate the start of a new job. A job that requires relocating may also be out of the question, because it would necessitate changing doctors. Couples fear they would have to begin the medical protocol again. Sometimes magical thinking further clouds the work picture; people sometimes imagine that a new job would somehow affect their fertility, for better or for worse.

Over the years, infertile women have been advised to leave their jobs in the hope of enhancing their fertility. Unfortunately, this unfounded advice is another example of the myth that stress causes infertility, and is based on the assumption that work is stressful. In fact, work is sometimes the only respite when one is infertile. And, in reality, few occupations are known to have a negative impact on fertility. Some of the known exceptions are: work that involves dealing with hazardous waste; work that involves frequent travel (thereby preventing well-timed intercourse); and highly active occupations such as dance or professional sports, which may interfere with ovulation.

In our work, we encourage couples to try to keep their infertility and their career as separate as possible. Frequent doctor's appointments usually force patients to tell their employers that there is a problem, but they need not go into details nor feel obligated to keep others up-to-date on the nature and progress of their treatment.

We recommend, also, that couples speak with their physicians about the time that is likely to be involved. While the course of treatment cannot be predicted, a doctor can address such issues as flexibility of office hours, punctuality, and the time required for certain diagnostic tests and treatments. Patients feel less overwhelmed by the time involved if they can anticipate it and plan their work accordingly.

Being at a standstill in their desire for children, there is no reason why couples should put their careers on hold as well. We encourage infertility patients to consider ways in which they can enhance or enliven their work experience whenever possible. For some, this means additional schooling; for others it means starting their own business; and for most people considering a change in their work life, it means a different job. In addition, we remind couples that they will probably want or need to continue working once they are parents—that work is an extemely important source of gratification in many people's lives. Thus the years of infertility, though demoralizing, can also be a time of positive and creative career development.

There is yet another unfortunate way in which infertility interferes with one's career. Work that involves frequent or daily contact with pregnant women, babies, or young children, can be especially painful to men and women experiencing infertility. For example, pediatricians, obstetricians, obstetrical and pediatric nurses, day care workers, and preschool or elementary school teachers, are among those professionals who are especially vulnerable when infertility strikes. Their job, rather than being a respite from fertile family members or friends, becomes another dreaded place from which they cannot easily escape. Work that was once a source of pleasure, becomes a constant reminder of their sadness and lack of fulfillment.

In this chapter we include an essay and a poem by two women whose infertility has an impact on their career in different ways. Marilyn Santiesteban approaches this serious subject in a lighthearted way. Her essay illustrates a dilemma many infertile women face—they are attempting to move forward in their career life, yet they cannot make long-range plans. Their work life is on hold until their infertility is resolved. Reverend Theresa Mason's poem, "And," captures the sad irony of a woman whose chosen career necessitates repeatedly blessing those who have been fortunate enough to "be fruitful and multiply."

But I Could Be Pregnant Any Minute!

Marilyn Santiesteban

If you saw me on the street, you would classify me as one of those yuppie working woman types: thirtyish, Rolex watch, smartly tailored suit, Reeboks, sleek designer leather briefcase. You would expect to see me in the airport of any large city; in the financial district of Boston, New York, Chicago, or San Francisco; or in the boardroom of large corporations. But the place you'll find me most often is in the waiting room of infertility specialists. I look like an achiever, the sort of woman who gets what she wants. And that's true, except in terms of motherhood. Over two years of trying hasn't gotten me any results. Thousands of dollars of testing reveal nothing wrong, so I could be pregnant any minute.

My job requires that I travel a lot, making presentations to large groups, and generally representing my company. Clothes have always been an important part of my image. So I was surprised to open my closet and notice my clothes were looking a little threadbare. It was a shock to realize that I hadn't bought anything new in two years. Why bother investing in clothes I soon won't be able to wear? I could be pregnant any minute.

I drink hot coffee carefully so it won't hit the nerve of the cavity I've been putting off having fixed—after all this time, I'm pretty adept at it. You've heard the stories about how pregnant women's teeth go to pot—well, I thought I'd wait and get all that dental work done at once, since I could be pregnant any minute. Every year that passes seems to add another thing to the list of required repairs.

Looking at my calendar as I schedule meetings requiring travel, I notice the months are thickly peppered with cryptic notes reminding me when I expect to ovulate, when I need to take Clomid, when I need to go in for my HCG shots, plus my many doctor's appointments and RESOLVE meetings. There aren't many free dates. With the air travel guide listing all flights in the continental U.S. by my side, I calculate whether (if I get up *very* early), I can have sex, catch the 7:00 A.M. shuttle to New York City, have my four hour meeting, and still be home in time for my 4:30 A.M. post-coital exam. I wonder whether the pressure change in planes disrupts the cervical mucus? Oh well, I'll be pregnant any minute and won't have to do this any more.

At lunch time, many of my colleagues go off to the health club next door to exercise. I used to do that until my membership ran out a couple of years ago. I didn't renew it because they don't have a good prenatal program, and I could be pregnant any minute.

Instead of going to the gym, I work through lunch and have a sandwich and an apple (can't afford to get fat!) at my desk. I plan to take off extra time after the birth of our child, so my work has to be in tiptop shape. I glance at the calendar . . . if I got pregnant this cycle, the baby would be born around our anniversary. What an auspicious time! Of course, I thought I would be pregnant for our last two anniversaries, plus the last two Christmases, New Years, Easters, Valentine's Days, Independence Days, Labor Days, Memorial Days, Groundhog Days, and Arbor Days. Each one seemed to have a special significance. But I could be pregnant any minute, so I settle down and work twice as hard.

My boss calls me into her office. "You've been doing wonderful work," she tells me. "I would like you to consider this new position. It would mean travel and a more hectic schedule, but it's a big promotion. I'm pleased to be able to recognize your contribution." I am surprised to be offered this promotion, since I've turned down the last two offers I've had.

I smile and thank her, telling her I'll think about it. I know she is puzzled that I don't jump at the chance—it *is* a terrific promotion—but I just don't think I can accept when I could be pregnant any minute.

I take the commuter train between home and work. There's always a large crowd packed on the platform waiting for the train. Today is no exception. Suddenly some burly construction worker squeezes in right next to me and lights up a cigarette. I turn to him and rage, "Can't you read?! Smoking is *not* allowed down here!" I guess I'm convincing—he immediately puts out the cigarette and mumbles an apology. I could be pregnant! How dare he put my child at risk from passive smoke! In two years, I've never let anyone smoke near me.

While commuting home, I start thinking about dinner. Since I rarely have time to cook during the weekdays, coordinating nutrition and the amount of time I have is no small feat. I mentally review the menus in the takeout places in my town. Food that's good for you always seems to cost twice as much as food that isn't. Until I started trying to get pregnant, I would eat any old thing. Now I'm a lot more careful. I'll be glad I ate healthy foods—I could be pregnant any minute! Besides, the staff at my regular places know me quite well by now, and can anticipate what I will and won't eat.

What I *should* be doing on the train ride home is looking over this college catalog. I need to take a few extra computer classes to really be up on the technology I work with every day. It's hard enough to coordinate my medical needs, my work needs, personal needs, and the stress of two long years of waiting. I can't handle another thing. Besides, who wants to be hugely pregnant, trying to squeeze into those school chairs? Or waddling across Harvard Square? Not me, and I could be pregnant any minute. I stuff the college catalog into the deepest recesses of my briefcase.

At home I kiss my husband hello. While I take care of dinner, he asks me what kind of wallpaper I would like in the living and dining rooms. We've been in our house over a year. Time enough to start making changes to reflect our personality, rather than that of the previous owners. But I want to start with the "extra" bedroom—the baby's room. Over the last two years, I've planned that room a dozen times. First I thought I would do it in primary colors and wallpaper bordered with balloons. Then the TV show "Dynasty" spawned a whole new look with brass cribs and lots of lace. Lately I'm leaning towards sturdy oak antiques. I haunt the baby furniture places. I know exactly how long it takes all the furniture, wallpaper, and curtains to arrive. I could be pregnant any minute. I dreamily consider this while my husband extols the virtues of neutral colored grasscloth.

Later as I read the paper, I particularly notice names. I have a mental list of favorite names. They've changed over the years to reflect my current preferences. I ask my husband how he feels about Paige for a girl and Matthew for

a boy. "Don't you think you're rushing things?" he asks. I smile indulgently.
Men! I could be pregnant any minute.

In the bathroom as I prepare for bed, I see the unmistakable red flag of
infertility. It seems I won't be pregnant any time soon, after all.

"And"

Theresa Mason

"What are joys and concerns?"
the visitor asked, with his eyes twinkling.
"Things that concern you such as health or situations in the world,
Things that you are happy about," I replied.
"Then," he replied, almost bursting out of his seat,
"Sharri and I are going to have a baby!"
They held each others' hands and glowed in the joy.
I had known they were pregnant.
She had called me twice that week.
I had recommended the gynecologist
Who I see for infertility.
Sharri had moved here recently
But, I had known her from a previous church where I had been pastor.
I had only spoken to him on the telephone, in returning calls to her.

I saved the prayers for them and their baby
Until the end of my pastoral prayer and finally prayed
"For Tim and Sharri and their baby."
But I couldn't stop there,
Because Chris six months pregnant
And Rick, and Devon their daughter, were sitting right in front of them.
Chris in her sensitive way,
Aware of my infertility
Had struggled over the best way to tell me
Five months before, that she was pregnant.
So I prayed "for Chris, Rick, and Devon and their baby.
But I couldn't stop there because Cheryl and Dan
Absent that day, were just as far along as Chris and Rick,
And I knew it was a tough pregnancy for her.
So I prayed "For Cheryl and Dan and their baby."
In my struggle for words
To pray for these three families,
I paused with the preposition:
"And"

Sharri and Tim and their baby,
Chris and Rick and Devon and their baby,
Dan and Cheryl and their baby,
                    And . . . . .
That "And" loomed giant
Grew larger than the prayer for me
Carrying with it the emptiness inside my womb
And tied me to John.
I dared not open my eyes and glance towards him.
My head buzzed with their names
and threw a silent plea to God for us
That our names be added to the list.
And debated making that prayer public.
It seemed like an eternity.
It was
In spite of my barrenness
what you call
"a pregnant pause."
My hand clenched the pulpit
Knuckles white,
As I tried to transfer the tension in my throat
To keep my voice from breaking
In praying the good news.
But the silence ended.
Somehow, with my hand gripping the pulpit
And my heart pleading its silent pleas to God,
I found my voice to keep the pastoral prayer going.
My words stumbled around about new life and love
And God's Spirit with them,
Until I managed to take it to the end with a phrase leading
into the Lord's Prayer.
I sat down after the prayer
Grabbed for John's hand as the liturgist prepared for the offertory,
with the same hand that had clenched the pulpit.
He held my hand gently and I held on tight
To prevent the tears from welling up.

Later in the afternoon while running on the track
The tears came.
While exercising on the monkey bars
My swing caught up short
And I fell to the ground landing on that same hand
It stung from the rocks beaten into it and bled.

6

Infertility and Religion

"Be fruitful and multiply"

S INCE biblical times, organized religions have emphasized the importance of bearing and raising children. With baptisms and brises, bar
mitzvahs and communions, religions celebrate the births and rites of passage
of their children. Most religious holidays are joyous occasions. They are a
time to renew one's faith and to celebrate life. Holidays, too, mark the
passage of time and the continuity of the life cycle. Religious holidays, particularly Christmas and Hanukkah, tend to focus on the young, involving
them in prayer and song.

There is no comfortable place in organized religion for the childless couple. They have no one to take to an Easter Egg hunt, and no small child to
ask the four questions at the Passover Seder. For most couples, even ones
who do not consider themselves observant, religious holidays are usually
painful. At the very time when they feel most in need of the comfort and
support that their religion might offer, they find themselves left out and
alone.

Individuals find that infertility affects their religious beliefs and obser-
vances in a variety of ways. For some, infertility prompts a major "crisis of
faith." They search their pasts for reasons why they are being punished. If
they find something, then they have a way of understanding their suffering.
Others, confident that they have not transgressed, feel betrayed. Believing in
a "just and merciful God," they question why they have been abandoned,
and why others seemingly less deserving, have been blessed with children.

But not all of those experiencing infertility feel a loss of faith. Some report
a deepening of their religious beliefs. Although they feel left out on religious
occasions, they find that in exchange, they are spiritually strengthened. For
them, God acts in "strange and mysterious ways." Though they have not yet

discovered the reason, there must be a purpose to their suffering. A purpose, not a punishment, might ease the pain.

For others, infertility creates a different sort of religious dilemma. Many were born into families that embraced a particular religion, but chose, for whatever reason, not to continue that tradition. Infertility revives old questions and conflicts. Some couples who consider themselves atheists or agnostic, discover that they feel more of a religious identity than they thought. These feelings are most apparent when they are considering adoption, surrogate mothering, or donor insemination. These individuals are often surprised to find that the religious background of a birth or donor parent matters to them—that they feel a basic connectedness to those of their faith.

The importance of fertility, and the anguish of infertility, dates back to the Bible. Rachel cried out to God, "Give me children or I die." Her words echoed the pain of Sarah, Leah, Elizabeth, and others who were all infertile. But for these women, prayers were answered. Though they suffered the pain of childlessness, they eventually bore children.

Today infertile men and women know all too well that prayers are not always answered. As they begin to consider the alternative means of conception now available to them—in vitro fertilization, gamete intra-fallopian transfer, surrogate mothering, and donor insemination, they discover new ways in which their religion of origin can have an impact upon their infertility.

"Be fruitful and multiply" is central to the Judeo-Christian tradition, but some religious leaders do not support their member's efforts to find new routes to parenthood. Catholics considering the new reproductive technologies are confronted with opposition from the Vatican. They, like Orthodox Jews, are left with the difficult task of reconciling conflicting values, and determining what takes precedence—their religious beliefs, or their desire for a family. Both religious groups promote family life, but limit the methods and means of procreation.

For most people, religion is a connection to extended family. They may not go to church or synagogue, they may not say confession or light sabbath candles, but they do gather with relatives on many religious occasions. These holidays offer families an opportunity to catch up, renew relationships, and reminisce.

Family celebrations are not the same when a family member is infertile. Relatives cannot completely enjoy watching their nieces and nephews, or grandchildren, open presents on Christmas morning, when they are aware that a family member longs for a child. Similarly, the merriment of children searching for the hidden matzoh, on Passover, is dampened by the sorrow of the childless couple. And, at some family gatherings, there are no children. An aging couple waits for grandchildren with whom to share the festivities, while their children, the potential parents, are filled with sadness.

In working with infertile couples who have been religious, and are currently feeling conflict about their religious beliefs, we acknowledge that shifts in religious feelings or observance are common. Often it helps to talk with a sympathetic clergyman. Many of them, while supporting the doctrines or laws of their religion, may differ from the mainstream as to how to interpret these laws. When considering alternatives that may be frowned upon by more conservative clergymen, it can truly be a relief to discover that a religious leader of one's faith is supportive of a couple's "extreme" efforts to conceive a biological child. For those couples who seek more religious involvement, and who feel left out of family oriented holidays and celebrations, we suggest exploring new ways to express their religious feelings. For example, one infertile Jewish woman wrote a memorial prayer for unborn babies, to be recited during the memorial service on Yom Kippur. A Christian couple found meaning in serving meals to the homeless on Christmas Day.

In the pages that follow, Rabbi Michael Gold presents a personal and theological account of what it means to be "Infertile, Male, and Jewish." Lisa Shearer Wilkins, in her letter to the Pope, voices the dilemma that many Catholics feel in the face of the Vatican's reaction to the new reproductive technologies. And finally, in "Prayerem" (half prayer, half poem), Jean DeMers Gilroy asks God to deliver her from the agony of infertility and make her feel whole again.

Infertile, Male, and Jewish

Michael Gold

I am a rabbi of a traditionalist bent. I am also an infertile man, and the adoptive father of two beautiful children. These various aspects of my identity have colored how I view marriage, how I view masculinity, how I view fatherhood, and how I view God.

When my wife and I were married, we agreed that we wanted a large family. We spoke about four children. Our only disagreement was how soon to begin. I was ready to try to conceive a child immediately. My wife believed that a couple needs at least a year to work on their marriage before seeking pregnancy. I realize now that she was right, yet little did I know that all those birth control pills would be wasted. We both had medical problems that precluded our getting pregnant, at least without intensive medical intervention.

Still, that first year was important. Jewish tradition sees two major purposes of marriage. The primary one is companionship and the secondary one is procreation. In my counseling I have seen too many infertile marriages break up. Too often one partner seeks someone who can give him or her a baby that the other partner cannot provide, resulting in adultery, divorce, guilt, and blame. I have come to realize that no couple should ever pursue the procreation part of their marriage until they have put time into the companionship part. Thank God, my wife and I did that. Our marriage was in a position of strength to pursue first intensive medical treatment, then adoption.

After one year, we threw the birth control pills away and began our quest to have a family. We assumed that it was automatic, the next step in a smooth continuum of school, courtship, career, marriage. Several months went by and nothing happened. Our doctor said, "Relax, don't worry. These things take time." Our friends and my congregants were beginning to wonder why a rabbi's wife was not pregnant already. We were becoming more and more depressed.

Finally, with the strong suspicion that something was wrong, we set up an appointment at a major infertility clinic in New York City. Like most men, I assumed that they would find some medical problem with my wife, do some surgery or give her some hormones, and we would have the baby we desperately wanted. After all, wasn't infertility a woman's problem? Reflecting this bias, traditional Jewish law (halacha) frowns on sperm tests, and permits them only as a last resort. When the doctor recommended a sperm test for me, I reluctantly agreed to it. She then came back with the news: my sperm count was so low and my sperm quality was so poor that there was no chance my wife could get pregnant.

My mouth fell open, and my wife started to cry. Our infertility was my problem. It took several years to realize that infertility was neither my problem nor my wife's problem, it was *our* problem, and as a couple we would solve it. All that would come later, though. For the moment, it felt like the doctor had impugned my very masculinity, and told me that I did not have what it took to do the number one thing men are made for—sire a child.

Early on, we turned to religion for whatever comfort it could give us. There is a saying that the purpose of religion is "to comfort the afflicted and to afflict the comfortable." We felt afflicted, but there seemed to be little in traditional Judaism to comfort us. We read the Biblical stories of God punishing a woman by closing her womb. We read the Talmudic law requiring a man childless after ten years to seek another wife with whom to fulfill the mitzvah of "be fruitful and multiply." We read modern responses calling artificial insemination by donor an abomination and in vitro fertilization immoral. We felt betrayed both by God and the long rabbinic tradition that claims to speak in His name.

Unfortunately, I was viewing Judaism very superficially. Since then, I have put a great deal of time and research into exploring those strands in the Jewish religion that can comfort and support an infertile couple. I have even written a book on the subject. For example, infertility in the Bible is usually not a punishment but, on the contrary, an affliction of the most pious. Abraham and Sarah, Isaac and Rebecca, Jacob and Rachel, Elkanah and Hannah, among others, were all unable to conceive, yet they are models of God-fearing individuals in the Bible. What struck me is that none of them passively accepts their infertility. They pray, they seek intervention of holy men, they try a surrogate mother arrangement, they adopt. The lesson of Judaism seems to be that passivity is not a virtue; I do not need to accept my infertility as God's will and do nothing.

As for the ten year limit on a childless marriage, I noticed that it historically fell out of practice. Jewish tradition seems to place greater importance on the love, companionship, and permanence of marriage, even if that marriage has no children. I noted the rabbinic story of a childless couple that divorced after ten years of marriage, and celebrated that divorce with a party. The husband, slightly drunk, told his ex-wife "Whatever you see in this house that you want, take with you." He then fell asleep, only to wake up in his wife's parents' home. She told him, "You said that I could take whatever I wanted. Well, I wanted you." Marriage is much too important to be destroyed by infertility.

As for the rabbinic rulings on the forbidden nature of unconventional medical techniques, I found little to support these in Talmudic literature. Take artificial insemination by donor. Many rabbis (not just orthodox) had forbidden it. Yet, the Talmud explicitly states that a child conceived in a bathtub is legitimate, and the mother could even marry a high priest. The midrash says that Ben Sira was conceived in precisely this way. The ancient law of Levirate marriage sets a precedent where one man's seed is used to conceive a child in the name of another man. There seemed to be room for a permissive ruling on donor insemination and other new techniques of conception, particularly when a mitzvah (divine commandment) as important as "be fruitful and multiply" was involved.

Most important, my exploration of Judaism taught me that our affliction is not a punishment from God. The book of Job made clear millennia ago that there is no direct causation between our sins and our suffering. My wife and I knew that we were good people and would make wonderful parents. Obviously it was not going to be easy for us. Infertility is a loss and we needed time to mourn. But there is also a limit to mourning and a time to act. Judaism teaches that if the world is not perfect, our job is to perfect it.

Here is where a strong marriage helps. My wife and I were each other's best friends, and we decided that we would do whatever it took to have the child we wanted. We would try surgery on me. If that did not work, we would consider artificial insemination by donor. Our next step after that would be to pursue adoption. Our goal was a child; we were less concerned with how that child entered our family.

I went through two rather extensive surgeries that laid me up for the good part of a summer. They were partially successful, and our hopes were raised again. Yet still my wife did not become pregnant. Soon, she began a series of tests. To our dismay, we discovered that she had hormonal imbalances, and that it was unclear whether she was ovulating. Now it was her turn for drugs, daily thermometer checks, and finally surgery. Still, there was no pregnancy. The medical option did not work for us, though we have not given up on someday achieving pregnancy.

At the height of our medical treatment, we received the most exciting phone call of our lives. A teenager was pregnant in the south, and her attorney was searching for the right adoptive family. Were we interested? An immediate decision was needed. A number of thoughts occurred to my wife and me as we discussed the issue. Could we afford it? Were we giving up on pregnancy? How could we explain it to our parents, who still had no idea about our infertility problems? Yet, we knew these opportunities are rare. We said "Yes," and two months later our son, Natan Yosef, entered our lives.

As we brought the baby home, we knew that there were issues that must be faced. Most important, the baby's birthmother was gentile, requiring that he have a formal conversion. When our son was four months old we did a symbolic circumcision, immersed him in the mikvah, and gave him a

Hebrew name. We then celebrated his arrival with a huge kiddush in my congregation. Three years later we did the same thing for the arrival of our daughter, Aliza Chasha.

The adoption of our two children was the most wonderful thing that ever happened in our family, not only for my wife and me but also for the four grandparents, the various uncles, and other relatives. No child could be more loved in our family. Yet, once again, Jewish tradition had little to say that could guide us.

In exploring Judaism, we discovered that there is great emphasis on biology. Even now, when I chant the grace after meals and come across the part where I bless "myself, my wife, and my seed," I cringe. These are certainly my children, but they are not my seed. My son, now five, has spoken as young children are wont to do about marrying his sister. I tell him that it is forbidden, although I know that by Jewish law it is permitted. After all, they are not blood relatives. In fact, by Jewish law even their conversion was conditional upon their accepting Judaism at the age of majority. I know that at thirteen my son can protest his infant conversion and retain his gentile status. I assume that with a good Jewish education, he won't. I know that traditional Judaism has laws of guardianship but not of adoption. There is not even a word for adoption in classical hebrew. ("Imutz" was coined by modern Hebrew lexographers.) All of these laws are based on the importance of biology in Jewish identity.

Once again, I have explored Judaism on a deeper level, searching for strands of the nonbiological. There are beautiful statements of the teachings such as "The one who raises a child is called the parent, not the one who gives birth." For me, one of the most meaningful rabbinic teachings states that if one finds the lost object of one's father and one's teacher, the teacher's is returned first. If one has a choice of rescuing or redeeming a father or teacher, the teacher comes first. To quote the rest of this teaching: "For the father only brings a child into this world, the teacher prepares him for the world to come."

I have reinterpreted this in a modern idiom that makes sense to me. Given a choice between being a progenitor or being a mentor, the mentor takes priority. It is more important to be the one that raises a child and passes on one's values to that child than merely being the sperm donor. I have decided that in Judaism, masculinity is ultimately proven not by siring a child but by raising and teaching that child.

It is for this reason that I have become totally comfortable with adoption as a way of building a family. Others, particularly men, have asked me, "How can you love a child not your own?" My answer is always, "The minute you hold them in your arms, they become children of your own." It has nothing to do with biology. I realize that my children have a biological identity separate from me, and I hope to share as much about that identity with them as I can. Yet, they are "my" children: given my name, my religion, and my values.

As strange as it sounds, there are times I thank God for my infertility. I believe that it has made me a better husband, a better father, a better man, and a better Jew. I am a better husband in that I have realized what is most important about my marriage. To quote a term in the marriage blessings, my wife and I have become "reim ahuvim," loving friends. Our companionship, our intimacy, our helping each other cope, have become central to our marriage. We have also become partners, working together to bring children into our marriage and to raise them.

I have become a better father in that I have realized that the essence of fatherhood is not biological but spiritual. I have become a better man in realizing that infertility has nothing to do with masculinity. It is unimportant whose seed created these children; what is important is whose love will sustain them.

I have become a better Jew in that I have confronted my tradition and found those strands that can give me comfort and strength. I have found the traditions that reject passivity and see me as God's partner in perfecting the world. I have found the traditions that would condone aggressive and even unconventional medical treatment to conceive a child. I have found traditions that reject biology as the only source of parenthood and rather allow for spiritual parenthood. Finally, I have found those traditions that see God not as a source of punishment, but as a source of strength in coping with adversity.

I look at my children and I truly see the hand of God. They could have easily been aborted like thousands of others, or borne into families who were not able to properly love or care for them. Something moved two very different birthmothers to carry these pregnancies to term and to go ahead with an adoptive placement. And something led these two children to my wife and me. Some may call it luck or fate; I believe it is the hand of God. Other infertile men have lost faith; my infertility has made my faith stronger.

Vatican Adds to Isolation

Lisa Shearer Wilkins

Dear Pope John Paul II,

Because of the Vatican's recent ruling on artificial means of conception, I now find myself an alienated Catholic; a member of that new "immoral" group—infertile people. Pronouncements such as the one you have recently made seem to serve only one purpose: to add an additional hurt to a situation that is already marked by incredible pain, isolation, frustration, loneliness, confusion, and helplessness.

Infertility is not something a couple would choose to have happen to them. In fact, the idea of bearing and raising children is something most people take for granted. It is assumed that we are all fertile and that when we decide to start a family it is as simple as going off the pill. Pregnancy will soon follow. For many of us, it simply does not work that way. My husband and I have desperately wanted a child of our own for more than four years now. It is quite possible that the only way we will ever have a biological child is by using what you call artificial and immoral means. My reaction to this decree is one of anger and deep pain. The experience of infertility seems to be absorbing my whole life right now. This is a time in my life when I most need comfort, understanding, and love. Yet the Church invariably labels my efforts to have a family as immoral, and refuses to support me and my husband in our quest for a child born to us.

The Vatican has said that no couple has an automatic right to a child, yet we do have an automatic right to seek medical attention for diseases, accidents, and illness. In fact, many of these diseases and illnesses are what cause infertility. You say we should just heed God's will and accept our fate in life. If the Catholic Church believes in a God who arbitrarily wished infertility or any other such tragedy on people, then I have a hard time believing in such a God. God gave men and women incredible talents to use. And many people have used their God-given abilities to create medical technologies that help infertile couples. To ignore these "gifts" would be to laugh in the face of a God who expects His people to use the knowledge He has bestowed on them to help other people.

I have heard comments not only from you, but also from other active Church members, that our extreme efforts are acts of selfishness, and that it is really not up to us to decide if we are to be biological parents or not. One of the responses to infertility that bothers me most is when we are told we can always adopt. Adoption is not the easy process it once was. Many people wait three to four years, often longer, for babies. The expenses associated with adoption, as well as infertility care, can be a financial hardship for many couples. Adoption agencies investigate every detail of a couple's life. They are the ones who decide if you are to receive a child or not—not God. If everyone had to go through what adoptive parents have to, it is likely that many would be turned down as parents.

There is not a day that I don't think about infertility. It permeates every aspect of my life. If you or anyone else who is so quick to judge my efforts, could catch even a glimmer of the pain I feel each month when my body once again reveals no sign of life, then perhaps some compassion might fill your heart, and you might understand why, in our love, we would go to extremes in order to create a child together. I want to bear life and will probably never understand why this tragedy has happened to us.

I have tried to become more vocal about my infertility. My hope is to raise people's awareness that the pain of infertility is real, and as devastating as any life crisis can be. I want to let people know that what we need is support and understanding, a patient heart and a listening ear. Criticism in regard to our efforts to achieve a pregnancy only serves to alienate us more. I am hurt by your pronouncements about infertility, but mostly I am saddened by the fact that the Church and her people are so quick to judge and label, rather than be what I think Jesus has asked each of us to be: compassionate, loving examples of himself.

Sincerely,
Lisa Shearer Wilkins

Prayerem

Jean DeMers Gilroy

Lord, take me back or forward
To a place where broken shards of joy
No longer cut me when I try
To piece them back together
Into the fragile whole
That not so long ago
Was my life's ardent dream.

To a time without the joylessness
That settles on perception
Like the long Icelandic winter

My sun will never rise.
They say to be your parallel
Should be my vision's healing.
Your suffering had constituents;
Mine rings in empty rooms.

I've hit the wall of my humanity.

Father, (they say you are one
So you know from where I'm speaking)
Grant me this intervention,
Or I beg you in your mercy,
Let me no longer care.

7

Pregnancy Loss

P REGNANCY loss is a common occurrence. One out of every five or six pregnancies ends in miscarriage. In fact, the rate may even be higher because sometimes a miscarriage occurs so early that a pregnancy has not yet been identified. A miscarriage is almost always unpleasant, both physically and psychologically. But for those couples who long for a baby, particularly after having experienced infertility, or a previous pregnancy loss, it is an extremely painful event, remembered long after the physical ordeal is over.

Approximately 75 percent of all pregnancy losses occur in the first trimester, usually as the result of an abnormal embryo or an implantation problem. Late pregnancy losses, occurring between the thirteenth and twentieth week, are usually caused by problems in the attachment of the fetus to the placenta or uterus. They can also be caused by structural abnormalities in the uterus or by an incompetent (weak) cervix. Other less common causes of miscarriage can be multiple pregnancies, the contracting of a serious illness or infection during pregnancy, or exposure to hazardous chemicals.

Another much more serious cause of pregnancy loss, is an ectopic pregnancy, a situation in which the fertilized embryo implants itself somewhere other than in the uterus. Most commonly, the tube becomes the locus of attachment, but ectopic pregnancies have also occurred in various locations in the abdominal cavity. Ectopic pregnancies are usually found sometime early in the first trimester, as the woman experiences increasingly sharp or severe pain in her abdomen. If the problem is discovered early enough, the tube can often be saved, but immediate surgery is necessary to remove the embryo. If the tube ruptures, it not only impairs her future fertility, but worse, it can threaten her life.

The chances of miscarriage increase with age. As a woman approaches her late thirties, the statistics grow larger, as more medical problems potentially develop. Sometimes deficiencies in certain hormones can cause a miscarriage, and treatment may then involve hormone therapy. After three or more miscarriages in a row, a woman is referred to as a "habitual aborter."

Miscarriage often comes as a surprise, particularly to couples who had little trouble becoming pregnant. Most couples have a sense that a positive pregnancy test means they will have a baby. When they miscarry, they are stunned by the experience. Couples who have been infertile are more prepared for this eventuality. They have grown accustomed to loss each month, and may believe that they will never bear their own child. Nevertheless, they have been hoping for the best, and perhaps, in their most optimistic moments, they did believe they would have a child. A miscarriage transforms their lingering fears into a painful reality.

The first signal of an impending miscarriage is usually blood. Bleeding, or spotting, however, does not always mean the pregnancy is over, or even in trouble. Sometimes bleeding has nothing to do with the condition of the fetus. In fact, half the women who experience some bleeding in their first trimester will go on to bear healthy babies. When bleeding does signal a miscarriage, it may occur just before the miscarriage or well in advance of the actual event. Usually, some cramping or discomfort occurs as well. When a woman is actually miscarrying, especially if she is further along in her pregnancy, she may have severe cramps or even contractions, as the uterus is expelling the fetus. Other signs of miscarriage are often noticed in retrospect. Women who had experienced nausea, usually begin to feel better. Or their breasts may cease to be swollen. They may feel more energized. In short, at some point before the miscarriage occurs, they begin to lose their symptoms of pregnancy.

Everyone reacts differently to loss. Yet most people experiencing a miscarriage, no matter how early in the gestation it occurs, feel some measure of grief. The nature and degree of this grief may be determined by various factors, including a prior history of infertility; previous pregnancy losses; and other major losses in one's life, such as the death or serious illness of a parent. Grief is often related to how late in the gestation the loss occurred. In general, the longer the pregnancy, the greater the grief. When a couple has been infertile, and then miscarries, the pain is enormous and the grief prolonged.

Perhaps what is most difficult for couples experiencing miscarriage, is that they usually receive little recognition or validation for their grief. Others do not seem to understand that the fetus or embryo was very real to them—a developing person about whom they formed many fantasies. They may have even chosen names for it. Worse still, people, in their attempts to be reassuring, often make unhelpful comments such as, "It was all for the best; the baby would have been deformed," or, "At least you know you can get pregnant." Couples rarely feel relieved after a miscarriage, that they are being spared the expense of a defective child. Their fantasy was about having a healthy child and their pain is about that loss. Furthermore, couples who have experienced long-standing infertility do not know they can get pregnant again. They fear that their last pregnancy was a random event, never to be repeated.

A miscarriage can be a real jolt to a woman's physical self-concept. Women who regarded themselves as healthy and physically fit may view themselves as seriously damaged, unable to perform the "simple" task for which their body was designed. For women who have been infertile, a miscarriage simply reinforces these feelings. They can not produce or carry a baby. They may feel unwomanly or even asexual. Certainly the experience of a miscarriage perpetuates their feelings of being out of control.

In addition to affecting one's physical self-esteem, miscarriage can also have a devastating effect on one's emotional well-being, especially if infertility has rendered her even more vulnerable. Often physicians do not know why a particular pregnancy ends in miscarriage, and so there is no specific reason they can give their patient. And this uncertainty makes it easier for the victims of miscarriage to blame themselves. Guilt often prevails over rationality. Women search their minds for what they must have done wrong. Perhaps they shouldn't have jogged their usual three miles? Maybe they didn't eat enough protein the previous week? Or even worse, perhaps they should never have had sexual relations the other night? The truth is that none of these events caused their miscarriage, but sometimes it is easier to blame oneself—and have an explanation—than to feel out of control.

In addition to guilt, women who experience pregnancy loss often feel angry and depressed. They may be angry at the world in general, or angry at God, for allowing the miscarriage to have occurred, particularly if they had previously been infertile. Anger can often be turned inward, leading to depression, especially if guilt is prevalent. But when friends and family can truly empathize with the couple's grief, the couple can usually recover more quickly.

Another reason why the grief of pregnancy loss can be so prolonged, is that there are no formalized rites or rituals in our culture for saying goodbye to a nonviable fetus, that was indeed so real to its potential parents. Recently, however, some couples are beginning to devise their own ceremonies for that purpose. They may do it privately themselves, or invite close family and friends to share their grief. Some couples actually bury something that symbolizes their "child" to them. In this way, their loss becomes more tangible to the world, as well as to themselves, and helps in the grieving process. Symbolically, they can bury the past—not forget it, but put it aside—and move on, with renewed strength, to face the future.

Rituals can help, and so can family and friends. Nevertheless, it is important to recognize that grieving a miscarriage can be a very long process. Couples involved in this painful event have experienced a death—the death of their potential child, who had just begun to be formed. For infertile couples, a miscarriage is an even more complicated and difficult experience. A confirmed pregnancy enables them to move one big step beyond their infertility. Yet a miscarriage plummets them back into despair to face the stark reality that they still have a long way to go before their dream is realized.

In the following pages we include two poems and four essays. In "Guenever Loses Her Baby," Wendy Mnookin conveys the anguish of a historical figure, Guenever, desperately hoping for a pregnancy, whose period arrives ten days late. In "Learning to Live with It," Pamela Matz describes the increasing pain and emptiness she experiences after three successive miscarriages, and the toll it has taken on her marriage. In "Nature's Hoax: The Story of an Ectopic Pregnancy," Paulette Bodeman chronicles the events surrounding her ectopic pregnancy, which became a medical emergency. Both Ray Noll and Sandy Van Wormer speak about the anguish of late pregnancy loss. The former buried his daughter, a "successful" IVF attempt, at eighteen weeks' gestation. The latter describes the all-encompassing grief she still feels, six months after her daughter was born dead, at twenty-one weeks' gestation. Finally, Barbara Crooker in her poem "Stillbirth" captures the pain and everpresent memory of the child lost years earlier that she never got to know.

Guenever Loses Her Baby
Wendy M. Mnookin

3 days late

Is it possible
  after all the years
    of filling space
with emptiness
  that a child
    latches on
and grows
  stretching the shell
    of my body
around her
  molding me
    to mother?

5 days late

I'll have a feast—
  light all the candles
    drape the banners
serve sixteen courses
  and a board of pastries
    minstrels will play
acrobats tumble
  and at the end
    a horn will sound—
"I'm
  with
    child!"

8 days late

Those who hate
  Arthur and me
    will watch her closely.
Green eyes or gray?
  Red hair or brown?
    Which one does she resemble?
Maybe me—
  her mother's child
    exposing no one

leaving me
  always uncertain
    whose child she is.

9 days late

I can't bear
  the days of waiting,
    not knowing.
What if
  she looks
    like Lancelot?
I must talk
  to my ladies
    find out
what to do
  how to shake her
    loose.
No!

10 days late

I dream
  I m a wild duck
    flying
Arthur
  sends his hawk
    to bring me down
I'm grabbed
  by the neck
    twisted
a whistle
  I fall down
    and down
I can't fly
  I drop
    to the ground
broken
  the dog's mouth
    closes on me
he brings me
  to his master
    Lancelot
I wake to blood.

Learning to Live with It

Pamela Matz

In September 1985, Norman and I began trying to have a baby—that is, I put away my diaphragm, which, for many people I knew, was all it took to conceive. I was thirty-seven, Norman was thirty-eight; we had lived together for a year and been married for five months. I had had an abortion when I was twenty-two (I got pregnant despite a Dalkon Shield) and another when I was thirty-five. The roads each of us had taken, and the road we'd been on together, to feel capable of bringing up a child, had been long and hard.

When we didn't conceive after six months, I began taking my morning temperature. So, it's not quite so simple, I thought. But a few months later, I had a positive pregnancy test. The anxiety of not conceiving ended. And the whole world seemed vibrant and accessible to me, as if a light had been turned on, or as if everything I saw had suddenly come into focus. We both knew that you weren't supposed to count on a pregnancy until after the first trimester. But miscarriage had never happened to anyone close to me, and the danger did not seem real. The fact that I had little nausea or fatigue I attributed to my unambivalent attitude. (I've found out since, that, to the contrary, morning sickness often signifies a successful pregnancy—another irony).

In my eighth week, I discovered one morning that I was bleeding and I went straight to the clinic of the university where I work. A doctor told us that the ultrasound showed no heartbeat, that the embryo must have stopped developing at least two weeks before, and that I should have a D&C immediately. We kept asking whether there was any chance the pregnancy could be saved, whether we should wait to be sure before we had the D&C, whether there was any way to learn what had gone wrong, and to stop it from going wrong again. No, no, he said, this was just one of those things that happened, tests wouldn't show anything. The best—the only choice—was to have an immediate D&C. Six hours later that pregnancy was over, and the mourning started.

Shortly afterward, my grandmother had a stroke that devastated her, and when she died, two weeks later, it seemed a mercy. But with losing her I lost the chance to show her a great-grandchild, born to me. The kitten we got because we needed something young to love spent a week in intensive care

in the animal hospital and almost died. We had other accidents and sick-
nesses in both our families. It began to feel that everything we set our hands
on would go wrong. I dug into our house and had to be forced out, except
to go to work. I didn't want to see anyone who asked anything of me—even
to listen.

Norman and I stayed together, but it seemed as if, for a good stretch, we
didn't like each other much and we weren't much use to each other. In retrospect, I can unravel it: my sadness scared him. He felt he had to take care of
me, but what I asked him for—either to leave me alone or to be there with
me in the place where it hurt so much—he couldn't do. He couldn't leave me
alone because who can watch a loved one in pain and not try to help? And
he couldn't be there with me because that way of handling pain wasn't his
and, besides, we had never both lost control at the same time. So I was angry
at him for letting me down, and he was angry at me for putting him in a no-
win situation where he felt he had to deny his own sadness. And we were
both angry at each other because together we had lost our baby.

And making love? Making love had been the source of this misery. We
were both terrified of it happening again, of a second miscarriage. There was
no way to be light-hearted or naughty, and neither of us had much energy.
Each cycle, I would begin taking my morning temperature—and part way
through the cycle I would stop.

After ten months or so I succeeded in keeping a temperature chart for a
whole month, and the next month, we agreed, we would begin trying to
conceive. This meant making love according to schedule, when for months
we'd hardly been making love at all. Not surprisingly, we couldn't. First I
couldn't carry a baby, I thought, then I couldn't conceive, then my husband
and I couldn't even make love. When I eventually connected with a counselor, I told her I was at the end of my rope.

We did learn to make love again, but with a different heart for it than the
way we'd begun. We thought of making love by the temperature chart as a
difficult task we'd try to get through together, and that was all. No expectations of passion or sensual delight. And that April, I got pregnant again.

This time we told only one or two friends and we kept reminding each
other it was too soon to be certain of anything. At six weeks, almost exactly
a year after the first miscarriage, I began bleeding. I was able to persuade an
obstetrician about whom I had heard good reports to see me that day. A
series of blood tests over the next week showed what my feelings had
already told me—that I had lost the pregnancy.

The second miscarriage happened ealier in the pregnancy. My body had
changed less, I'd had fewer of the pregnancy feelings, I'd had a shorter distance to travel to get back to "normal." And, of course, this time we had

known from the very beginning that miscarriage was possible, that for some people, pregnancy is tentative.

We had had a three-week vacation scheduled in Italy and hadn't had time to cancel the reservations; so, soon after the miscarriage, we went. When I got my period again, in our room in a pensione in Florence, I cried the night through, cried for the two babies I hadn't had because of miscarriages and the two babies I hadn't had because of abortions. Norman woke and comforted me sometimes, but most of the night he slept. We'd learned some things about managing sorrow between us. And in the morning, we went on, and the next day was all right.

On our return, we went through the standard battery of tests, which turned up nothing. From my reading and talking to other women, I wondered if luteal phase defect might be a cause of the miscarriages. The obstetrician, though respectful of our concerns (and that mattered), advised that, since tests had shown me perfectly healthy so far, we should just keep trying.

All my life I had thought that having children was something that happens naturally *unless you prevent it.* But at this point I began to believe that having a child—biological or adopted—would happen for us *only if we consciously willed and worked toward it.* This is not the worst thing that can happen and people have gone through it and come out on the other side. But sometimes it feels as if there's a well at the center of the world we don't get to drink from. And sometimes I hear a voice inside me saying what fills me with rage when other people say it: that it would be all right, if only I could relax, if only I didn't care so very much, too much.

I transferred my care to a reproductive endocrinologist, who diagnosed a border-line luteal phase defect and prescribed treatment with progesterone. I also began seeing an acupuncturist, who treated me for strengthening of menstrual and reproductive functions, and who gave me the warmth and sympathy for which I felt starved. One month later I got pregnant. The doctor and the acupuncturist were delighted. Norman said this time he'd believe it when he saw the baby. I thought maybe this time it would be all right, but I tried not to let it show, not even to think it, hoping not to tempt fate. Then, as suddenly as a cloud covering the sun darkens a day, in the seventh week, depression hit me. Three days later my first ultrasound showed that the embryo was smaller than it should have been. A blood pregnancy test showed my hormone level was not rising appropriately.

I stayed home from work for five days. I felt as if I were sitting up with someone who was dying, except what was dying was inside me. Finally I had heavy bleeding, and cramping more painful than I'd felt before; I passed what I knew was pregnancy tissue, and it was over.

We were able to have a chromosome analysis of the tissue (which is not always possible) and were told that the pregnancy had not been genetically normal, could never have developed into a baby. That knowledge has been a relief, in a way I can't explain. During the pregnancy, deep inside my mind, I'd given a name to the baby. After we got the results of the genetic test, I felt able to take the name back.

After the third miscarriage, I felt my life had to change, that I could no longer live covering up or denying the pain I felt. I have taken a half-time leave-of-absence from my job. Norman and I are in a group for couples with infertility problems—that's painful, too, but it helps, I think. I've started some of the projects I always meant to do but didn't have the time for—from cleaning behind every appliance in the kitchen to thinking about writing a novel. I am acutely aware at moments that it is a miracle any of us are here at all.

It's four months later, and we have just started trying to conceive again. By now we've had every test that's ever been suggested to us, and the medical reality of our situation remains ambiguous. There's a good chance, we're told, we can have a biological child. How good is good? And how do we factor in my "advanced maternal age"? We may have other treatments. We are also thinking about life without children, though that's difficult for me to do. Wanting a baby seems rooted in my body. And we are going to information meetings at adoption agencies.

I am also—without knowing whether it will make any difference—staying away from my video display terminal (VDT); drinking bottled spring water; avoiding caffeine, alcohol, sugar, and processed foods; exercising; continuing acupuncture treatments; and learning to meditate.

I watch myself, and in quiet moments I see how much of my life now centers on the absence of a child. I buy things I don't really need; I turn on the radio, the television, the record-player, to make sound; I turn small encounters into emotional events, to fill the emptiness. And the emptiness doesn't go away. The lesson I am learning is not the one I looked forward to, the day I put my diaphragm away, but it is useful: when emptiness is what you have, you have emptiness to make your peace with.

Nature's Hoax:
The Story of an Ectopic Pregnancy

Paulette Bodeman

I was not overly concerned with the fact that my husband had a vasectomy several years prior to our marriage. It is a fact that many people in second marriages must deal with. We discussed our desire to have children together and decided that he would undergo a vasectomy reversal.

We were fortunate in that the surgery went well. We learned, however, that with most reversals, the optimal chance for conception is within the first few months following the surgery, for as time passes it becomes your enemy. With time, the sperm develops antibodies that make it impossible for the sperm to penetrate an egg, thus resulting in infertility.

Twelve weeks after my husband's surgery, I made an appointment for a check-up. I felt slightly crampy, was spotting, and I feared my endometriosis was flaring up again. Discouraged, I explained how I felt as the doctor examined me. He asked for a urine sample, and said to meet him back in his office. I thought his request odd because he never required a urine sample before.

A short time later we sat in his office and he beamingly announced, "I am extremely pleased to tell you that you are a few weeks pregnant." I could not believe what I was hearing! My head spun and I could not suppress a giggle. The entire staff knew of our attempts at conception, so consequently they took pleasure in congratulating me.

What timing! It was our anniversary, and I was struck with the thought of how perfect and precious a gift my announcement would be. We had a lunch date at one of our favorite outside cafes, and I risked being late by stopping off at a department store to buy a pair of baby booties. My voice shook as I asked the sales clerk to wrap the box in anniversary paper. I felt as though I were watching myself from a distance. Could this truly be happening? Will I wake up and discover that this is only a dream? But I carried the carefully wrapped package, placed it on the seat next to me, and tried to convince myself that this was real and that we had won the battle with endometriosis and a vasectomy.

I spotted my husband at a corner table and I greeted him warmly as I handed him the tiny package. As he opened the box I found it impossible to take my eyes off his face. The look of wonder quickly turned to surprise and joy, and instantly we were both crying and laughing and hugging, while people at nearby tables began to smile and stare. But we were oblivious to all but our own world that would soon include a little one.

The next few days were such a high for us. We called our family and friends, and revealed our auspicious news, then reveled in the wishes and love they sent in return. We also looked forward to our annual spring/ anniversary event where we spend a lazy weekend hidden away in a mountain cabin. It's a time devoted to enjoying good food, concentrating on each other without the distractions of everyday living, and appreciating the majestic beauty that surrounds us.

Sometime during our weekend getaway, I developed a dull pain in my lower abdomen, and my skin felt sore and hot to the touch. I wondered if the food was too rich or whether I was beginning to experience morning or afternoon sickness, but it was nothing like I had heard or read about. I did not even feel a little bit nauseous. The pain would suddenly be there, intensify, then quickly disappear. In the far recesses of my mind a chill of fear crept in, but I deliberately forced it back. Despite my growing discomfort we enjoyed ourselves. We anticipated the grand finale of our special weekend. Out of town friends surprised us with a visit and we were to meet them for dinner on our return home. We were anxious to tell them our good news.

As we were getting ready to go out, the pain in my side stayed for longer periods of time and the dull throbbing intensified into a sharp, stabbing sensation. My husband suggested we call the doctor, but I refused to admit it could be that serious, and I hated the thought of bothering him at home on a Sunday evening. I felt sure the pain would go away. We went to dinner, but our joy was clouded with our growing anxiety. I could not eat and we cut our visit short.

The pain continued until finally my husband insisted I call the doctor. Another physician was on call and I felt uneasy discussing my symptoms with someone I did not know. He was vague, yet sympathetic. I was not bleeding so he did not think I showed signs of miscarriage, and he suggested if the pain persisted to call my doctor on his return the next day.

When night slipped into day I wearily crawled out of bed and tried to analyze my pain; it had become familiar. Looking down at my belly it appeared larger than the day before. Could I be showing already? Now along with the pain, and fear, was growing confusion. What was happening to me? I felt hungry and thought that must be a good sign. We had an early breakfast together, and when my husband left for work I began changing the bed linens. While tugging at one corner, a sharp pain stabbed in my lower left side and took my breath away.

I knew I was about to be sick, and staggered to the bathroom. I collapsed on the cold tile floor and could no longer force the fear from surfacing. I began to sob. I have never been so ill, or so unable to control my body or my emotions. The next several minutes I spent either draped over the toilet bowl, or seated on it. I could not believe this was happening.

Was this a miscarriage? Still there was no bleeding. I knew I needed help, but all I could think of was my husband. I needed him. As I crawled to the phone the pain became so unbearable I passed out. When I came to I was more frightened than ever and that motivated me to reach the telephone and dial his office. When I heard his voice, my defenses crumbled and I sobbed, "Baby, something's wrong. I'm really sick. Please come home." I later learned that he made the usual half-hour drive in fifteen minutes. When I saw the look of terror on his face as he held me in his arms, I realized the danger I was truly in. He contacted my doctor who agreed to meet us in the emergency room.

The walk from our bedroom to the car was almost impossible to make. I was in so much pain he could not carry me, or touch me. I shuffled, bent over, clutching my side, and every few steps I sunk to the floor trying to catch my breath and the will to go on.

The emergency staff were expecting me and efficiently lifted me out of the car and placed me on a stretcher. My doctor was not there yet so we waited anxiously for him. Before long he was examining me and told us that he suspected I was trying to pass a kidney stone. He ordered an ultrasound and I prayed that he was right. A cousin of mine had passed a stone while she was pregnant and everything turned out just fine.

I wanted to scream out in pain as they placed the tabs on my belly. My husband still held my hands and murmured words of love and reassurance. We watched the screen not really knowing what to look for when the intern blurted, "I thought you said you were pregnant?"

"I am."

"Well, I don't see a fetus here."

"What do you mean you don't see a fetus; what's that supposed to mean," I angrily snapped.

The doctor knew she had handled the situation badly and tried to apologize. She simply said, "I'm sorry, you'll have to discuss this with your doctor."

They wheeled me to my own room and I was given something for the pain. My husband and I barely spoke. Both of us were drawn into our own circle of fear, pain, and sadness. And still he held my hands and continued his litany of love.

Finally my doctor arrived and explained I had suffered an ectopic pregnancy, and had lost my left tube. Through ignorance and desperation I clung to hope. "Is the baby all right?"

He looked directly at me and asked, "Don't you understand what I'm telling you?"

I shook my head no. "I've never even heard of ectopic pregnancy."

He then further explained. "The embryo implanted itself in your left tube and began to grow there. But soon it grew too big and it caused your tube to rupture. And with it you are bleeding internally." He proceeded to explain what he must do, and why, as he tried to prepare me for the forthcoming surgery. I welcomed the release from pain it would bring, and tried not to think about my "baby."

After surgery the drugs allowed me to block out reality and any thoughts of the demise of my unborn child. But as the day drew nearer for my release, the dosage of drugs was lessened, and with it, came remembrance. I tried placing my hands on my belly as though through love and sheer will, I could put the embryo back in its proper place, where it would mature and grow into a healthy living baby.

My mother flew down to help care for me and many days I cried in her arms. I knew I frightened her with my uncontrollable grief and despair. She was unsure how to talk to me and how she should react to the crazy, wild things I would say. We have a close relationship and never before have we had difficulty communicating, but this time we reached a stalemate. I tried to explain to her and to my husband that I felt as if my child had died. They in turn, tried to understand, but they could not. They both were struggling with their overwhelming relief that I had not died, and fear that it could happen again. My mother in her love for me, told me that it really was not a baby, not even a pregnancy, but an abnormality, and that I must think of my health and getting well. And my husband, caught up in his own sorrow about our loss, and his fear of losing me, did not know what to say.

During my mother's stay, I allowed myself the security of hiding within the walls of numbness. But after she left, I got terribly depressed, and although my aching body slowly healed, my aching heart did not. I often looked down at the red livid scar slashed across my body, and was filled with self-loathing and disgust. I felt my body had betrayed me, and that I was not a whole woman. I wondered how my husband could still love me and I felt sure God must have punished me. I asked myself what I had done wrong. I replayed each day in my mind, trying to remember, seeking an answer. I was filled with anger. I not only disliked myself, I disliked the world. I wanted to lash out and hurt others the way I was hurting.

Eventually the doctor told me we could try to conceive again. Though I only had one tube, he felt sure I could get pregnant easily. He did not mention that one tube cuts your chances in half, or that when you have had one ectopic pregnancy, the likelihood for another is greater.

I was filled with terror at the possibility of a reenactment, but I became obsessed with the idea of conceiving again. My husband and I argued. He did not want me to risk my life again, yet I concluded that he did not care about having children. The strain on our marriage was severe, but we did continue trying to conceive.

After six months of attempts to conceive, I became disheartened. I was ready to move on and see a specialist. I found books and articles concerning infertility and read everything I could. I no longer felt ignorant of my own body, and at the mercy of others. We have now spent two-and-a-half years with our new physician. I feel confident in him; he is a warm, caring, concerned human being.

At my husband's suggestion, and with encouragement from our doctor, we sought marital counseling. Through these sessions, we began to explore our feelings about our infertility and the impact it has had on our lives. We have gotten closer again in the process, and though I feel resolved about the past, I will never forget the "child" that was with us for such a short time.

The years since the ectopic pregnancy have been filled with pain and sorrow, but also with self-discovery. We now know, however, what is truly important to us. We want to raise a child together, to give and receive love, to teach and to learn. And this experience does not need to come to us through biologically creating a child. We know that we can create the family we want through an alternate plan—through adoption. We are currently awaiting placement. And we will gratefully accept the gift of love a birthmother will give us.

Deserted Cities of the Heart Revisited

Ray Noll

January 9th, 1987. I buried my daughter today. She lived eighteen weeks inside her mother's womb, a joyous miracle of science, conceived in a laboratory through in vitro fertilization. Yet she was part of our love and desire; now this field of tall grass contains her. A dream child who carried our spirits high above the years of grief and hopelessness. The others had passed on as buds in a late frost, but her bloom was so close to opening with new life. She gave us strength and an optimism that fueled our flagging energies and discarded ideals. With her passing, so much has been lost.

I dug the grave deep, to keep her safe from the packs of feral dogs running hungry through these suburban farmlands—the only protection I could ever offer her. I capped it off with a heavy piece of carved slate. Her mother looked on, transparent white from loss of blood, her tears frozen into scarf folds. Her red-blonde hair, now a graying crown, blowing over the hill of empty trees. The winter sun sat low in the sky, sharpening us into long shadows edgy with despair. The cold brilliance seemed fitting. This child was our radiant union, her light was our future vision. We became lions again in a country looking backwards.

Our friends and family encircled and embraced us, weeping in the dry grass. Incense burned, words of consolation from tight throats were uttered, and pink miniature carnations were individually placed on her small stone. Her cedar casket settled softly into the sienna sands of a vanished ocean.

Now, at night, the bed shudders with the deep sobbing of a mother robbed of her joy. Her full breasts are now lumpy with milk that has no place to go. Her rounded belly so recently squirming with life is only a distended uterine cavity, healing in the aftermath of forced labor. Still too fresh in her mind are the wondrous nights of feeling the baby's movements through her fingertips, the sweet internal conversations she would have with it. How she reveled in her shape as her body swelled with a new promise. All replaced by mournful longings. "I want my baby back. I wanted this baby so much. I feel so dead."

I am broken and humbled. I wanted to be changed by her birth; instead I am transformed by her death. She taught me about the fragility of life in the angry face of the world. I find myself only interested in creating life-affirming images, images of compassion and introspection.

It is a familiar place, our uneasy truce with grief. The years change numbers, the feeling remains, surging worse with each loss. All my dead, unborn children, united as laughing stars in the night sky, my friends forever.

For you can only measure your joy by the depth of your sorrow.

Late Pregnancy Loss: When Reality Becomes a Nightmare

Sandy Van Wormer

It is very difficult to write this story since it has been only a short time since we lost our daughter, Brittany, delivered stillborn at twenty-one weeks. I am hopeful that writing something in her memory will help me heal and begin to move on.

My pregnancy ended very suddenly. I had had an infertility problem for the past three years and then a first trimester miscarriage, but these difficult experiences had been followed by a successful pregnancy and the joyous birth of our son, Colin. When I was pregnant again, a little more than a year later, and my first trimester passed uneventfully, I assumed that my problems were behind me.

An incompetent cervix. That was the diagnosis that my doctor gave me as we rushed into surgery in an effort to save my pregnancy. He would attempt to perform a "cerclage," a procedure that meant sewing my cervix shut so that I might carry to term—or at least long enough for the baby to survive. As it turned out, I was already dilated ten centimeters and the amniotic sac was almost completely out of my uterus. My doctor performed the surgery but my water broke and the baby had to be delivered. She weighed 11 ounces and was 9½ inches long: stillborn.

Stillborn. The word sent chills through me as I lay in bed, in shock and disbelief. I couldn't cry; I was numb. I felt like someone had amputated my legs. I dreamt that a nurse came into my hospital room after the surgery and said, "Sorry, Sandy, your legs are gone, and you can never have them back."

During that initial period of disbelief, I held on to the idea that it was all a mistake. Perhaps my baby was really still alive and the hospital had mistakenly taken her from me. Soon a nurse would bring her to my door and apologize. All would be forgiven and I would sing with joy. But this was not the case. My reality had become a nightmare.

We held a memorial service for Brittany the day after Christmas, two and one half weeks after her birth and death. I found the service to be particularly painful because it brought back the longing I felt to hold her in my arms. I had not been allowed to see her or hold her because she had been injured in delivery. I felt angry at the hospital for taking her from me without even offering so much as a picture.

Then I began to feel mad at myself. Why me? I must have done something to cause this tragedy. I looked to my past for a reason. In its absence I turned to God. How could a just and merciful God do this to me?

My grief was so powerful that it interfered with my ability to love and care for Colin, then twenty-one months old. He was still in diapers and each time I changed him, I was reminded of my other baby. All I had of her was a birth certificate with her footprints on it. I felt terrible that this piece of paper seemed to matter more to me than my young son, whom I loved and cherished and who had once been a source of such pleasure.

I decided that I was having such a difficult time because I was unable to cry. If felt as if I were swollen with sorrow. One day I sat down on my bed, took out all the memories that I had and waited for the tears to come. Eventually, I began to weep, then to sob for several hours. I was exhausted when it was over but indeed, the tension had been relieved. I began doing this daily for several weeks until I began to feel a little better.

Six months have passed and I remain depressed, angry, bitter. Often I feel numb and disoriented. I'm tired much of the time and have little pleasure being with other people, even those most dear to me. I'm frightened by the way in which my grief consumes me.

My husband tries hard to put up with me. I keep telling him to be patient, that I can't help the way I feel. I'm trying. He cried when we lost Brittany but he hasn't mourned as I have. He doesn't feel the pain and bitterness. I try to tell him how I feel, but sometimes I'm afraid to tell him because I find I feel hostile toward him. As with my son, it is frightening to feel that I've lost the capacity to love.

I'm told that it takes one to two years to mourn a baby. I keep reminding myself of this each time I take a step forward and each time I take two steps backwards. At my worst moments, when I fear that my grief will never end, I force myself to recall my relationships with loved ones, particularly Colin, before Brittany's birth and death. Comforted by memories of the good times, I wade my way through this thing called grief.

Stillbirth

Barbara Crooker

She said, "Your daughters
are so beautiful.
One's a copper penny,
the other's a chestnut colt."
But what about
my first daughter,
stillborn
at term,
cause
unknown?

Ten years later
and I sift the ground
for clues: what was
it I did?
Guilt is part
of my patchwork;
grief folds me up
like an envelope.

In the hospital,
the doctors turned
their eyes, told me
not to leave
my room.
But I heard them,
those babies in the night,
saw women from Lamaze
in the corridor.
They would be wheeled home
with blossoms & blankets,
while I bled the same,
tore the same,
and came home, alone.

Later,
women showered me
with stories
of babies lost:
to crib death,
   abortion,
   miscarriage;
   lost;
   the baby
   that my best friend
   gave up
   at fourteen.

They wouldn't let me hold her:
all I saw were fragments:
   a dark head,
   a doll's foot,
   skin like a bruise.
They wouldn t let me name her,
   or bury her,
   or mourn her.
Ten years later
and I do not have
the distance:
I carry her death
like an egg
in my pocket.

8

Half Biologically Ours: Donor Insemination and Surrogate Motherhood

COUPLES experiencing infertility usually view the problem as shared, hesitating to designate one partner or the other as "the patient." Nevertheless, there are many situations in which one person is found to have a significant problem and the other partner is most likely fertile. When treatment attempts fail, some couples frequently raise the question, is it preferable to have a child that is genetically half ours than not ours at all?

Many couples answer "No." The problem belongs to both of them, they reason, and the best route to becoming parents would be to adopt. Or, they might decide to live childfree. These couples reject the idea of having a child that is genetically connected to one of them and not the other. Other couples in this situation like the idea of raising a child who is genetically related to one of them, but they may have serious misgivings about the alternative reproductive choices that are available.

In this chapter we will discuss donor insemination (known as D.I.) and surrogate mothering. Although they are biologically equivalent, these procedures are very different experiences emotionally, legally, and financially. Furthermore, the effects on the children produced may be very different. Hence we will look at them separately, noting some of the commonalities but focusing primarily on the unique dilemmas and rewards involved in each experience.

Donor Insemination

No discussion of the non-medical aspects of donor insemination can occur without an examination of the meaning and impact of male infertility. A diagnosis of azoospermia (no sperm) or some other serious and untreatable male problem is inevitably a severe shock to a couple. It is often experienced by the man as a fundamental assault on his masculinity. Donor insemination, though a practical solution to the problem, does not diminish the intense feelings of loss experienced when a man learns he is unable to father a child.

Masculinity is an issue for men for most of their lives. Beginning even before adolescence, boys compare the size of their genitals. Later they exchange tales of sexual prowess. Power and potency are often equated with the size and function of their sexual organs, which in turn affects their self-image.

Men also have strong feelings about passing on their lineage, usually through their surname. Even though many women are retaining their names after marriage, most children are given the surname of their father. For men, probably more so than for women, the ability to genetically link one generation to the next, is a central component of parenthood. Rarely are girls named after their mothers, but our society continues a long tradition of *juniors* and *thirds* and *fourths*. Even though many men would not consider naming their child after themselves, they do sometimes maintain fantasies of producing a "chip off the old block."

By the time they approach motherhood, most women are very familiar with the frustrations and problems of their reproductive system. Most women experience some discomfort with menstruation, and many have suffered from severe cramps or premenstrual syndrome. Many women have had vaginal infections and almost all have endured the embarrassment of having a pelvic examination, usually performed by a man. And because things have not always gone so smoothly, women are probably more prepared than men, at least less shocked, when something goes wrong.

Men are far less familiar with difficulties related to their reproductive system. Occasionally a man will have a testicular infection or an injury that brings medical attention and concern to his genitals. Most often, though, men grow up assuming that successful sexual performance is an indication that their sexual organs are functioning normally.

Along with determining ovulation in the woman, a semen analysis should be one of the first steps in any infertility work-up. All too often, gynecologists overlook this simple procedure if they have discovered a problem in the woman. A semen analysis determines the number of sperm in the ejaculate as well as the percentage of motile sperm. The form of the sperm (morphology) and the number of abnormalities and anomalies present also offer important information regarding a man's fertility. The test itself is easy to do and can be performed in most medical laboratories.

For most men, a semen analysis is a very stressful experience. Although it involves none of the physical pain, precise timing, or expense of some of the female infertility tests, it raises serious concerns for men, as they must produce a fresh sample of sperm. Many report feeling embarrassment or shame at having to masturbate in the lavatory and ejaculate into a jar. Men are used to masturbating in secret, often believing that "real men" have "real sex" and that this act marks them as being an inferior male.

Poor results from semen analyses are jolting. Men who assumed potency, who spent years worrying about their girlfriends getting pregnant, may learn that they have no sperm. Others are told that while the count is good, the motility is very poor, which means the sperm probably won't go anywhere. Some men learn they have a problem that may possibly respond to female hormones or to surgery, but many are told that there is no treatment available for them. Progress has been slow in developing means for treating male infertility.

A diagnosis of untreatable male infertility is usually followed by mention of donor insemination. Sadly, men are rarely given the opportunity to mourn the loss of their biological child. All too often their physicians, wives, and even the men themselves expect that they would readily embrace the opportunity to have their wives impregnated by another man's sperm.

The decision to do donor insemination is not an easy one. However, those couples who do undertake the procedure usually do so after careful examination and soul searching, as there are a number of difficult and serious issues that need to be addressed. They include: secrecy; donor anonymity; donor selection; shared parenting; and sexually transmitted diseases.

Secrecy

For many years donor insemination has been a procedure shrouded in secrecy. Couples undergoing D.I. were usually advised by their doctors to tell no one—not even close family, friends, physicians—the circumstances of conception. Since artificial insemination is not a visible action, as is adoption, even the offspring produced need not necessarily know.

Couples undertaking D.I. today frequently challenge this doctrine of secrecy. They question what it would mean to have such a highly charged family secret beginning from conception. They worry about the strain they would feel among family and friends. They understand it would take an enormous amount of psychic energy to maintain the secret, particularly when comments were made about whom their child resembles. Couples wonder how they and others would react if the child had some distinctive feature different from both parents.

While many couples considering D.I. reject the notion of secrecy, most have serious questions about how much they should say—and to whom. They recognize that just as there are dangers in being too secretive, there can also be problems involved in telling. Many questions, both general and specific, come up for the couple considering donor insemination. For example, if one good friend knows, does that mean all good friends should know? Where do they draw the line? How do they decide who to tell and who not to tell? Will one person tell another? Couples are challenged to figure out how honest and open they wish to be, while still maintaining privacy and a sense of control over the decision and its ramifications.

Donor Anonymity

Related to the issue of secrecy is the matter of donor anonymity. Except in a few unusual situations when a couple arranges for a friend or family member to be the donor, the identity of most donors remains permanently unknown. D.I. programs maintain that this anonymity is essential in order to attract donors. Parents and professionals involved in adoption know that people have a need to identify their roots. With adoption, these roots are often traceable. Currently, most adoption agencies give their clients a good deal of information about their child's birthparents. This information can later help children search for their birthparents if they should choose to do so. The information itself can help the adoptee by being the basis of a more fixed and solid identity.

The D.I. child and his parents face a permanent blank space. Since no identifying data about the donor remains, there is no way that anyone can obtain information about the biological father. Though some programs are considering changing this policy, current practice is to maintain secrecy. Thus the sense of rootlessness, so often troubling to adoptees, can be even more profound for those children who are completely cut off from half of their genetic and cultural heritage.

In addition to unanswered questions about background and identity, donor insemination poses specific dilemmas regarding medical history. Although donors are reportedly well-screened, and families are sometimes given a little medical history, this history is vastly incomplete. It covers only up to the birthfather's young adulthood. There is no ongoing access to significant medical events that happened later in his life, or in the lives of his blood relatives.

Donor anonymity also raises fears and fantasies of incest. Living in a community where D.I. is a fairly widespread practice, and where a given donor can father several children, there is always the chance that two people with the same birthfather will mate. While this is unlikely in reality, it is a disturbing and powerful fantasy. Adoptees sometimes report feeling that they were unable to marry until they had identified their birthparents.

Donor Selection

Donors tend to be drawn from medical school classes or other graduate programs; intelligence is usually a given. In most programs, couples are assured that in all probability they will get a donor who is physically and emotionally healthy, and whose eye color, hair color, and stature match the husband. Still, couples worry. They worry that their child will inherit some unfamiliar physical or mental characteristic forever reminding them of the unknown biological father. Donor anonymity contributes to the sense of mystery and loss of control.

As in adoption, couples find that they often have strong feelings about the religious and ethnic background of the donor. Some couples are taken by surprise at the importance they place on having a donor of the same religion as the father, particularly if the husband or wife is not religiously observant. Identity becomes even more important when one is threatened with losing it.

No one knows to what extent personality characteristics and temperament may be inherited. Couples undergoing D.I. wonder about their donor's personality and whether their offspring will be like him. Since most donors are medical students, couples attach feelings that they have about physicians, in general, to the donor. Some are comforted by their belief that physicians are intelligent, caring, hardworking individuals. Others are troubled, believing that most doctors are self-centered, materialistic, one-dimensional people.

Shared Parenting

Couples considering D.I. worry that the husband will not have strong paternal feelings toward his child. Though they recognize that all men are left out of the pregnancy experience, they worry that these feelings will be more pronounced in their situation. They worry also that the husband's lack of involvement in the conception will carry over to his role as a parent, and that he will have difficulty bonding with their baby. Mostly they fear that the circumstances of their baby's conception will always be with them—that they will never feel the child truly belongs to both of them.

Couples express additional concerns about how donor insemination will affect their marriage, both during the procedure and later, if they succeed in having a child. Wives are often ready to attempt D.I. sooner than their husbands. Their desire for pregnancy is usually great. During the decision-making process, men often feel that their wives want a baby more than they want them. Husbands understandably feel jealous and rejected, fearing that their wives don't need them. Couples worry that this jealousy will intensify when a child actually enters the family. They fear also, that there will be conflicts about discipline, authority, and who really is in charge, and that the mother will always be regarded as the "real" parent, the one with ultimate authority.

All prospective parents share the nightmare that their child will have a terrible birth defect or a genetic disability. Couples involved in D.I. are particularly fearful. Wives worry that their husbands will leave them if there is something wrong with the child, since the child is "not his" anyway. Another concern is that the husband will withdraw emotionally, offering little or no support to his wife or child.

Sexually Transmitted Diseases

Living with the AIDS epidemic all around them, couples fear the worst: that they will contract this deadly disease. Programs attempt to screen their donors well, especially for AIDS, but also for other sexually transmitted diseases. It is impossible though, to eliminate all risk. Ironically, the former acronym for artificial insemination by donor—AID, closely resembled the acronym for acquired immune deficiency syndrome—AIDS. Because it was difficult to ignore this connection, the acronym AID was recently changed to D.I.

In order to guard against AIDS, many couples opt for frozen rather than fresh sperm, as it enables physicians to test for the presence of the AIDS virus. The odds of conceiving with frozen sperm, however, are not as good. Thus couples must weigh the odds for conception against the odds of acquiring a fatal disease, truly a life or death decision. And while AIDS is the most alarming threat, herpes and other veneral diseases are also of concern to the couple considering D.I. Even when real risks are small, worries can be substantial. Donor anonymity certainly contributes to a sense of feeling out of control, that one's life is in the hands of fate.

The Adoption Alternative

Before moving on to D.I., most couples take a serious look at adoption. Perhaps for the last time they weigh the equality offered by adoption, against the opportunity for a pregnancy and a child that is genetically linked to one of them. Once again they review their feelings of having a child whose biology will most likely be a mystery against the advantages of known "good genes." D.I. is certainly a more practical alternative. It is far cheaper than adoption and, if successful, the wait is not very long. No homestudy is required, and no time-consuming paperwork need be done. Though D.I. is more practical, many couples do choose to adopt, feeling that the emotional complications of donor insemination are more than they want to handle.

Some husbands initially resist donor insemination believing that for their wives, pregnancy is more important than their marriage. Often, when wives agree to adopt, husbands feel reassured that they are loved and needed. They then may choose D.I. or adoption. Such men see that their wives are indeed responsive to their loss, and are willing to share it.

The Procedure Itself

Those couples who do finally decide to use D.I. often find that the difficulties of infertility do not go away once the decision is made. While some encounter a straightforward process that brings prompt success, others embark on a long and complicated journey. Donor insemination, on the average, takes four to six months before conception occurs. Often it takes much longer, and couples must, once again, face month after month of heartache.

Some couples are inseminated by their physicians, while others go through a D.I. program. The latter involves certain medical tests, some of which may be repeats of ones done earlier, as well as interviews with a social worker. Just as the program heads must evaluate a couple's preparedness for D.I., the couple must evaluate the program for themselves.

In the past, a key question for most couples entering a D.I. program was whether to use fresh or frozen semen. As discussed previously, frozen specimens allow greater protection against sexually transmitted diseases. Also, some couples report feeling more comfortable with frozen sperm, regarding it as more of a medical tool than fresh semen, which can evoke feelings of adultery. In 1988, however, the American Fertility Society strongly recommended using only *frozen* sperm in inseminations. Thus fresh sperm would presently be difficult, if not impossible to obtain. Couples preferring fresh sperm would probably have to seek a known donor.

Once a couple is involved in a donor insemination program, other considerations arise. One of the chief complaints of women undergoing D.I. involves scheduling. Some large programs manipulate their patients' cycles so they all ovulate at the same time. Therefore, the program can be more efficient at what it does, since everyone will be requiring the same medical services at the same time. The timing of the inseminations may be convenient for the medical staff (no weekends) but very inconvenient for working women. Women who are inseminated by their doctors, or by programs that do not manipulate ovulation, often complain that the office is inadequately prepared for them if they ovulate on a weekend or a holiday. In most instances, they must agree to be inseminated a day or two early, or even worse, a day or two late, knowing that they have probably wasted their time and money.

Women undergoing D.I. raise complaints about other aspects of their treatment. Many are astounded by the insensitivity of some of the staff members, particularly with regard to issues of confidentiality. Some tell disturbing stories of planning for an intra-uterine insemination, only to be told that no one present knows how to perform this procedure. Women have occasionally been "forgotten" after an insemination—abandoned in an examining room, speculum in place, for an extended period of time.

All couples undertaking D.I. must make a decision about whether the husband will be present for the inseminations. Some couples feel strongly that it should be as much a shared experience as possible, and that the husband should, indeed, be "present at the creation." Others prefer to avoid dealing so directly with the stark medical procedure, and find it easier to have the wife go alone. And some couples disagree. The wife may very much want her husband's support and companionship, but he may find it difficult to be there.

Rarely mentioned in discussions about D.I. is the fact that men sometimes have fantasies about their wife "having sex with another man." While D.I. is clearly regarded as a medical procedure, there is often a sense between husband and wife, that the marriage bed has been violated. If the husband is not conclusively infertile, it is sometimes suggested to couples that they make love before or after the insemination, thus obscuring the absolute truth about the conception. Couples must decide whether they wish to be 100 percent certain about the conception, or whether they wish to harbor any doubts. In making this decision, they must also consider what action they feel would be best for the child that might be conceived in this way.

Finally, there is the question of effectiveness. While infertility patients will endure an enormous amount of inconvenience and pain to achieve a pregnancy, their best efforts do not always work. Artificial insemination, for unexplained reasons, does not work as well as sexual intercourse. Even when timing is "perfect" and all seems right, pregnancy still may not occur. Couples who struggled hard to decide about D.I. may feel profound disappointment when this, their carefully chosen alternative, fails them.

Despite all the problems inherent in the process, D.I. is a fairly easy way to create families for couples where there is a male infertility problem. Men who are able to grieve the loss of their biological children, and to confront feelings of jealousy, inadequacy, and rejection, most often do move on to fatherhood by donor insemination with ambivalent but generally positive feelings.

Surrogate Mothering

Among the various alternative reproductive technologies, surrogate mothering is probably the most controversial. Until late in 1986, surrogating was a quiet controversy. It was primarily infertile couples and perhaps some lawyers and clergy, who struggled with the complex issues involved. Then the Baby M case exploded into the media. By the time the case came to trial early in 1987, it was the focus of worldwide attention.

We have included both D.I. and surrogate mothering in one chapter because they are biologically equivalent. Each alternative, if successful, results in a child that is genetically related to one parent, but half of whose genes were provided by a donor. But because surrogating involves a *known* donor who carries the baby for nine months in her womb, and gives birth, it is a vastly different experience from its biological counterpart, D.I. Thus, these two alternatives raise very different psychological, legal, and ethical concerns.

Openness

As noted earlier, the secrecy and anonymity involved in D.I. are frequently a burden to couples considering this method of conception. Secrecy is not an issue, however, for couples using a surrogate, most of whom enter into open arrangements in which they know a great deal about the surrogate. On the other hand, with surrogacy, there are issues concerning contracts and custody. As everyone learned from the Baby M case, a surrogate can change her mind during pregnancy or after delivery, raising complex legal and moral dilemmas regarding custody. Although the local judge in the Baby M case essentially upheld the validity of the surrogacy contract, his decision did not establish a binding precedent. In fact, several months later, his decision was overturned by the State Supreme Court.

As of the writing of this book, the future of surrogacy remains to be seen. Thus, legally, the two biological equivalents—D.I. and surrogate mothering—are worlds apart. When a couple employs a surrogate, the wife must adopt the baby after birth; when a couple uses donor insemination, the infertile husband is legally the father from the time of conception.

Shared Parenting

Couples entering into D.I. and surrogate arrangements have different kinds of concerns about attachment to their unborn baby. While men often have powerful feelings of loss or rejection when their wives are impregnated by another man's sperm, they are, in reality, no more left out of the pregnancy and childbirth experience than they would have been if conception had occurred normally. Sometimes, however, the men anticipate they will have more difficulty bonding with the child when it is born. Sometimes their fears are founded, but most often, men form feelings of deep attachment sooner than they had expected.

Women are supposed to bear their children and deliver them into the world. They have nine months to emotionally and biologically become attached to their baby. In a surrogacy arrangement, though, it is possible that the husband/father will develop stronger feelings of attachment to the unborn child than will his wife, who is biologically left out of the experience. In most families, however, women are still the primary caretakers, so that adoptive mothers can anticipate bonding with their baby soon after it is born. Thus it is relatively easy for an adoptive mother in a surrogacy arrangement to fantasize about her role as mother, and to develop a feeling of connection to the baby another woman is carrying for her.

The Challenges

More so than with donor insemination, a couple considering surrogacy must anticipate multiple challenges within their family and within society. Couples using surrogates must understand that someday they will need to help their child sort out the unusual circumstances of his or her birth. Even when the surrogate recedes into the background, she is always psychologically present, as is the birthmother who surrenders her child for adoption. But unlike birthmothers in adoptive situations, a surrogate was paid to conceive, to gestate, and then to hand over her baby to another couple. The two situations have different emotional implications for the child involved as well as for the parents.

Couples entering into surrogacy arrangements must expect negative responses, including disapproval, from family and friends. They will surely be challenged by these reactions and may feel they must defend their actions. But for the infertile couple longing to be parents, surrogate mothering, with all of its problems, offers a potential solution to their infertility. For many couples, the opportunity to have a child that is genetically connected to one of them is important. For others, the appeal of surrogacy has less to do with genetics and more to do with control. Troubled by the randomness and uncertainty involved in adoption, they find the contractual process of surrogate mothering to be comforting. They like the idea that they will feel involved with their child from the time of conception, and may have some input into prenatal care.

Surrogate arrangements remove some of the uncertainty about timing that is characteristic of an adoption. Adopting couples often do not know if they will become parents in a week or in a month or in a year. Couples working with a surrogate have a much clearer time frame. They can plan their lives much easier.

Despite strong opposition on the part of many people, some infertile couples do make surrogate mothering their second-choice route to becoming parents. They struggle with all the questions about genetic inequality, as well as with the legal and ethical considerations. They worry that something will go wrong—very wrong—as it did in the Baby M situation. But essentially they feel that surrogate mothering is a reasonable means of becoming parents.

The Opposition

Those who oppose surrogate mothering, and they are vehement in their opposition, regard it as baby selling. They feel that those who pursue it are at best short-sighted, and that they are insensitive to the difficulties inherent in the situation. Despite the fact that, as a tradition, surrogacy dates back to the book of Genesis, opponents see it as creating a baby supermarket that threatens to destroy the very fabric of family life.

Opponents of surrogate mothering focus on what they regard as the best interests of the child. Rejecting notions that these children are created in love and given up primarily for idealistic or humanitarian reasons, they focus instead on the payment involved. They see it as destructive for any child to know that his biological mother was paid to conceive, carry, and give him or her away. They also raise concern for the surrogate's other children who must bear witness to the "selling" of their half brother or half sister. The half siblings are then deprived of having a relationship with one another, unless it is expressly written into the contract.

Opponents of surrogating focus also on the amount of money paid for this service, saying it promotes exploitation of the poor by the rich; in particular, women by men, as the latter hire the former to bear their children. While some accuse women of doing it for the money, others say that the payment involved is insultingly small, far below minimum wages. They note that in some surrogate contracts women are paid little or nothing if they miscarry, or if in some other way the pregnancy does not go as planned. Hence, there is some inconsistency in the argument regarding payment. If women are really doing it for the money, then why are they agreeing to such inadequate compensation?

Opponents of surrogate mothering argue more convincingly that those involved, particularly the surrogates, simply do not know what they are doing. They say that no one can give informed consent before birth, let alone before conception, and point to all that is known about the bond that develops between a woman and her unborn child. They remind us of all the women who planned to surrender a child for adoption and changed their minds at birth. They remind us also, of those women who have amniocentesis, intending to abort if the results are bad, and who then develop an attachment that precludes abortion or makes it more difficult. Finally, they add that a surrogate can have no way of anticipating the loss and guilt she may feel in the years that follow the surrender.

While they are critical of those who enter into surrogate contracts, opponents of surrogacy tend to voice their strongest criticism at those who promote these arrangements. They refer to them as "baby brokers" and regard them as scheming, manipulative entrepreneurs who have found a clever way to make money using people. They oppose efforts to legislate or regulate surrogacy, claiming that it should be outlawed instead.

Certainly there are compelling arguments on both sides of the surrogate debate. As clinicians working with infertile couples, we are well aware of the hope that this process can offer. But our experience with birthmothers and with adoptees has taught us that there is pain in both surrendering and having been surrendered.

We support legislation that will regulate but not eliminate surrogate contracts. Such legislation should remove or diminish some of the concerns that opponents have about the contracts and about the payment involved. Legislation offers the possibility of more equitable arrangements, including limitation of decisions that can be made before birth. In addition, proper legislation helps protect prospective surrogates and contracting couples from the "black market" that would inevitably develop if the process were outlawed.

Emotional Considerations with D.I. and Surrogacy

In working with couples exploring donor insemination or surrogate mothering, we encourage them to consider what it will mean to them to have a child that is biologically connected to one of them and not the other. We ask them to compare this option to adoption, which is most often their only alternative, and to try to determine which path to parenthood is truly better for both of them. Most important, we emphasize that in selecting D.I. or surrogacy, the couple must be in agreement; these options are too emotionally difficult for there to be any lingering sense that one spouse has pushed the other into something he or she was reluctant to do. It is also important that they agree on how private or secretive they will be in regard to telling others.

We ask couples to imagine their child at an older age, dealing with issues related to his or her identity. We ask them to imagine what their feelings will be and how they will respond to their child's concerns. We want them both to be comfortable enough with the alternative, so that they can agree on whether and when to discuss the issue with their child. We ask them to explore how they might feel if their son or daughter wishes to search for the missing birthparent.

Prior to actually following through with any of these options, the couple must grieve the biological child they could not produce together. Becoming a family through donor insemination or through surrogacy was not the original way they planned to become parents. The loss of a child who would have been a product of their combined biology is a loss that must be mourned. And when most of the grief has passed, they can move on to other alternatives.

We were pleased to discover that there were people who were willing to share their stories about donor insemination and surrogate motherhood, experiences that are often kept private, or not written about. We begin with Janie Sherman's humorous account of her travels with a large tank of frozen sperm, the contents of which she attempts to keep secret. Next are two more serious accounts of donor insemination. First, Stephanie Brigham poignantly reflects on how she and her husband dealt with the news of his sterility, and then chose donor insemination as an alternative means to parenthood. Then Michelle Parks in "Donor Insemination: The Gift of Life," offers thoughts of her son's conception and early years. This chapter ends with an enthusiastic essay by Tom and Barbara Pixton about how their daughter arrived via a surrogate mother.

As the Sperm Turns

Jane Sherman

There must be a law that women undergoing donor insemination will ovulate on weekends. Inseminations must be carefully timed to coincide with the release of the woman's egg, but doctor's offices are often closed on the crucial days of the month.

I was in this predicament one month, so I prepared a small ice bucket on a Friday morning, brought it to work, and called my doctor's office to arrange to pick up the semen. I was using frozen semen rather that a "live" donor. I knew that it had to be kept frozen until I was ready to use it, or the sperm would begin to die.

I had done this before. Once I got the semen home, I would put it in the freezer. On the proper day, my husband would inject the semen into my cervix, using a speculum and syringe provided by the nurse. This was anything but romantic, although it provided a real hands-on anatomy lesson for Charlie. But I digress.

Upon calling the nurse, I learned that the doctor had decided to allow me to take home the cylinder in which the semen was shipped from Michigan, to insure that the semen would not defrost. The nurse cautioned me that the cylinder was heavy, but I figured that I could manage to carry it for the fifteen minutes it would take to walk to my car.

Imagine, if you will, a rounded silver milk can, two feet high, with a handle at the top, and weighing approximately twenty-five pounds. Inside the silver metal exterior is a white plastic inner seal, containing incredible cold liquid nitrogen and three tiny semen samples in clear plastic capsules, clamped in a metal bracket.

As I lifted the cylinder in the doctor's office, I knew I was in trouble. I'm short, with a slim build. Gritting my teeth, I dragged the damn thing out of the building, resting every few feet. By the time I hit the street, I was sweating.

I was in downtown Boston, in the financial district, near my office building. As I staggered along the street with my unusual burden, I prayed that I wouldn't run into anyone I knew. Charlie, upon learning that I would be in this predicament, had asked me how I would explain what I was doing, should the need arise. Obviously, I couldn't just say that I was carrying the father of my children. I had assured Charlie that I would come up with some false but logical explanation when the time came, but I still hadn't thought of a good story.

Then it happened. "Janie! What's that?" It was Mary, a woman I hadn't seen in months, and she was staring at the cylinder with fascination. Oh shit.

"Hello there!" I chirped. "How have you been?"

"I'm fine," she replied, doggedly adding, "but what's that?"

Desperately, I offered the only explanation that came to mind. "It's something I picked up from a laboratory for a scientist friend of mine. He lives near me, and he asked me to do him a favor."

This story had more holes than Swiss cheese. There are no laboratories in the financial district, and the "scientist friend" theory sounded pretty lame. Nevertheless, I was committed to it now.

Predictably, Mary persisted. "But what's inside of that thing?"

Uh-oh. Now what should I say? "I don't know," I blurted. "He didn't tell me." Mary clearly thought I was dim-witted, but after a few more questions she gave up, and we parted.

Two blocks and twenty sweaty minutes later, three voices chorused in unison. "Janie! What's that?" Oh, great! Three coworkers were returning from their lunch hour. They were all examining the cylinder with interest, and one even started to lift it up and down.

Once again I offered the cockamamie scientist friend story. This time I even complained that my friend hadn't told me that the cylinder was so heavy, adding, with feeling, that when I saw him I was going to *kill* him. My friends were amused by my professed ignorance as to the contents of the cylinder, and started to speculate about what could be inside. One guessed that I was carrying a germ warfare experiment. Nuclear waste was also suggested. After a few more yucks at my expense, one of the three insisted on his carrying the by-now-loathsome article to my car.

Oh Lord. The car wasn't there. Charlie had taken it to pick up his relatives at the airport. When he returned with them, I would have to satisfy their curiosity too. In the meantime, I had to stash the cylinder somewhere, and I sure didn't intend to lug it into my office just to endure another inquisition. Thanking my friend for his help, I dragged the thing into the nearest bar. The bartender agreed to let me put it behind the bar counter for a few hours. I begged him to keep an eye on it, as it contained a "valuable scientific experiment." I was beginning to believe this myself.

I could tell you about finally getting home, and trying to find a time to do the insemination without tipping off the relatives who were visiting. This was complicated by a bedroom door without a lock. When, on Saturday afternoon, Charlie and I sheepishly said that we were going upstairs for a short nap, they probably thought we were planning a "quickie." We were—a quickie in a tube.

I wish I could end this story by telling you that a baby resulted from all the craziness. Instead, I must report that I have nothing to show for over one year of insemination attempts. Still, I have a loving husband as well as my health. For those I am grateful and, for the moment, they will have to suffice.

Playing the Hand You're Dealt

Stephanie Brigham

It was unlikely that the sperm count was actually zero. Because the test was probably done incorrectly, we were advised to have another. It also reported zero, as did the one after that.

Our decision to proceed with donor insemination was an easy one to make; it was either that or adoption. The adoption process seemed endless and hopeless. We would only turn to it as a last resort. And at my age of thirty-eight it was unclear an agency would accept us. Donor insemination would allow us to share the pregnancy and birth. Unlike couples with a low sperm count, we had no other hope and therefore did not have to agonize over other possibilities.

As we proceeded with the logistics of our decision—the doctors, nurses, therapists, and waiting lists—I felt hollow and empty, enthusiastic and hopeful. During the next year I became accustomed to feeling opposite emotions simultaneously. I had a long-term, constant, deep, and abiding sorrow that I would never bear my husband's biological child. I was surprised to learn that I had a picture in my mind's eye about what our child would look like, what features of his it would have, what characteristics of his it would inherit. All that was lost. For a time I couldn't look at him without breaking into tears. I would awake in the morning, see his profile beside me and slip into sorrow.

At the same time, there were lots of positive actions to take. There was excellent news concerning my fertility and we had every reason to expect success. But I still had erratic emotions. Taking my temperature every morning told me I was ovulating but also reminded me of our infertility: Up, down, Positive, negative, Happy, sad, Yin, yang.

My husband took the news much better than I. He experienced shock and regret; but he didn't have the ups and downs, didn't seem to experience the same bottomless sorrow. One day I asked him how he could simply accept the news and carry on with life in the new framework. His answer changed everything for me. First, he said one had to play with the hand one was dealt. Our hand was pretty good overall. How many tragedies had possible solutions, as ours did? Second, he thought of parenthood as two phases. The first was conception, which was an instantaneous roll of the dice. There followed a lifetime of love and influence in raising a child. All we had lost was the roll of the dice, we still had the lifetime. These words fostered a calm acceptance in my heart, and made me ache anew that this fine man would not be the biological father of our child. Up, down. Happy, sad.

On the eighth try our daughter was conceived. She is lovely, she is an angel, she is ours. Ironically, she looks like my husband. She has his gray eyes and a cowlick in the same place. The roll of the dice seems a long time ago. Now we are living the lifetime. Sometimes I still cry. But mostly we all laugh and coo.

Donor Insemination: The Gift of Life

Michelle Parks

When our son, Jeffrey, was a baby, the nurse in our pediatrician's office always commented on how much he looked like his dad. My husband and I would turn to each other and smile. I'm sure that when she saw us smiling, the nurse had no idea why her comment brought us such delight. She had no way of knowing that Jeffrey was conceived by donor insemination.

Looking back on our journey to parenthood, the decision to use donor insemination seems, in many ways, like the easiest part. If I concentrate, I can remember struggling with it and grieving the loss of our ability to have a child together. But with a diagnosis of azoospermia and with a strong wish to be parents, D.I. seemed like a good option—and opportunity.

Making the decision to try D.I. was easy; becoming pregnant by it proved very difficult. First, we learned that I did not ovulate. Then, with various combinations of Parlodol, Clomid, and HCG, I was able to achieve a "normal" cycle. We tried fertility drugs together with D.I. and eventually achieved pregnancy, only to lose it at eight weeks.

The miscarriage was extremely painful for us. A pregnancy that had been so hard to come by was lost. It felt as if there would never be another. Also, the process of becoming pregnant was exhausting to us. We had to drive three hours each day from our home in rural Vermont to our doctor's office in Boston. These trips were scheduled only a day or so in advance, so it became very difficult for us to be reliable at work. And the treatments themselves were unpleasant: a cold speculum, a plastic cervical cup, then a half hour on my back after the insemination. I remember lying there on the table and wondering if there would ever be any light at the end of this cold dark tunnel.

Then the light came. I was pregnant again and, this time, things went well. I remember being very anxious during the first trimester, but then relaxing once a heartbeat was confirmed. Once the pregnancy became real to us, my husband and I were able to share some of our thoughts and fears about its outcome. Would we have a child that looked nothing like us? Would we be able to love the child? Would something be wrong with the baby? How might he or she interfere with our marriage? We had a vague sense that some of our concerns were shared by all first-time parents, but wondered just what was a result of donor insemination.

We were awakened from our fears and fantasies about our baby by the reality of a very hard labor and delivery. I had medical problems and complications of anesthesia that resulted in a difficult and alarming high-tech birth. What a strange irony that I had equal trouble getting pregnant and "unpregnant."

When Jeffrey was a baby, my thoughts turned, at times, to his conception. I remember a recurring dream in which the donor appeared with a daughter named Susan. In reality, I knew little about him and had felt comforted by the fact that we lived far apart. I knew only that he was a physician, married and a father. I guess that his appearance in my dreams with his child, Susan, was my effort to make him real, to make sure that his life was complete, perhaps to differentiate him and his family from our own.

I have heard that couples considering D.I. worry that the father will not be involved with the child. That was not something that I was particularly concerned about and it has never been a problem. If anything, I think that our infertility and D.I. experience has made both of us more involved and enthusiastic parents. My husband takes great delight in his son, and Jeffrey, who worships his Dad, has already picked up most of his expressions and his mannerisms.

Jeffrey will turn four next month. This birthday, like those that came before it, will be a big occasion. We'll have a party for Jeffrey and his friends and then another for our families. At the family gathering, Jeffrey's grandmother will undoubtedly comment on how he has inherited her love of music; his uncle will talk about how Jeffrey is as curious as he is; Grandpa will reluctantly admit that "the boy is as stubborn as I am"; and all will agree that he got the best of his Dad and me.

In the midst of it all, I will probably take a moment to say a silent thank you to a man that I will never know. Though he must remain ever nameless and faceless, he is not forgotten. He gave Jeffrey the gift of life and he made all of us a family.

Becoming a Family: Our Experience with a Surrogate

Tom and Barbara Pixton

Our daughter, Catherine, who is now nearly two, was born to us by a surrogate mother. We are well aware of the controversy surrounding surrogate motherhood, but for us the experience has been a very positive one. It has made us a family.

Surrogate motherhood was the end of a long hard road for us. Barbara had two ectopic pregnancies, one of which was a frightening medical emergency. Then we tried IVF. It was an expensive, time consuming, physically and emotionally draining ordeal with little chance of success. We decided that before our emotional and financial resources were completely depleted, we had best move on.

Many people view surrogate motherhood as a means of having a baby that is genetically linked to one of its parents. For us, surrogate motherhood was simply a way of having a baby. We liked the idea that our child would be Tom's biological child, but that was not our primary reason for choosing this route over adoption. We chose it because we wanted a white, healthy infant, and from all that we had heard, this would be a difficult and lengthy process. Having had enough disappointment and enough waiting, surrogate motherhood seemed certain and more predictable.

Once we had decided to use a surrogate, we had to find an agency. We looked into a few different ones and decided on an institute in Kansas. It turned out that our choice was a good one—they were a pleasure to work with.

The process began with our selecting a surrogate. For us this was a fairly straightforward process. We weren't searching for someone who looked just like Barbara or who had Nobel Prize winning genes. We simply wanted a woman who was healthy, reliable, and who clearly understood what she was doing and why. Most of the women whose profiles were sent to us fit that description, but we kept finding that other couples had already contracted with them. Then we realized it was because the mail was so slow between Kansas and Boston. When we told the institute of our dilemma, they agreed to give us the first chance with the next available surrogate. And that is how we found Barb.

Barb is a happily married mother of five children. We knew as soon as we read about her and saw her picture that she would be fine. We signed the contract promptly and we began sending frozen semen specimens monthly. Since Barb had such proven fertility, we hoped that she would quickly conceive. But infertility had conditioned us well for the disappointment that we had to face once again: the frozen specimens apparently did not travel well. After six months, she was still not pregnant.

At that point we decided that Tom would fly to Kansas and produce fresh specimens. Fortunately, Barb not only has a very regular cycle, but she also predictably ovulates on Saturdays. Tom began flying out there one weekend each month for the insemination. On the third attempt she conceived.

We were so relieved that Barb was pregnant! We had begun to worry that she would become discouraged and would give up on us. The inseminations required her to take time off from work, and once she had to drive a long way in an ice storm. I guess that we were also beginning to feel that this experience, too, would end in frustration. When her pregnancy was confirmed, we felt that things had finally turned around for us.

We exchanged letters with Barb and she asked us to come out for a visit. At first we were afraid to become too attached to the pregnancy, but when she was seven months along, we decided to go, though we were somewhat apprehensive about the meeting. We feared they might not like us or they wouldn't appreciate Tom's sense of humor, or we would say something awkward and they would be offended. We feared we wouldn't have anything in common.

It turned out to be a great experience. We met at a park on a gray November day and as soon as we saw them our fears vanished and we felt as if we were meeting some long-lost cousins. We chatted for a couple of hours and then agreed to meet later at a restaurant. We liked her. We liked her husband. We had a chance to get to know their children and to see the way that they live. Our backgrounds and our lifestyles are very different, but we all got along well. We were especially glad to have met them during the pregnancy so that when Catherine was born we were not strangers.

We became very excited when Barb was in her final weeks and hoped that we would be able to be there for Catherine's delivery. As it turned out, we just missed it. We were staying in Philadelphia with Barbara's mother and phoning Barb every day. Being experienced in labor and delivery she had a strong sense of when the baby would come. She kept telling us, "Soon, but not today." When we finally received a call that she was in labor, we were on the next plane.

When we arrived at the hospital at 4:00 P.M. we found that Barb had delivered a healthy girl at 1:00 P.M. We were met by our social worker and immediately went upstairs to see Barb who was resting in bed and looked terrific. Her husband was watching a football game. Both looked quite nonchalant, as if this were something they did every day. Presently, the nurse brought in the baby and, looking around at the five of us, said, "Now, who would like to hold her?" Tom held her first and after a few minutes declared himself to be in "baby heaven!"

We were particularly touched by Barb's concern for our feelings. She had been worried that if we weren't there on time, there might be no one to hold Catherine, so she had asked if it was all right with us if she held her. We said, "Sure." Similarly, she had asked our permission before allowing the doctor, who was something of a "camera buff," to videotape the delivery.

The days and weeks after Catherine's arrival were a joyous time for us. At last a family, we celebrated with both of our families. Our mothers were particularly enthusiastic about their new grandchild. Our friends all knew what we have been through and they, too, were very excited. Meanwhile, we kept in touch with Barb and let her know about Catherine's growth and development and about the joy that she had brought us. We continue to keep in touch.

At nearly the two year mark, we have settled into family life and don't think a lot about how Catherine came to us. We do think about asking Barb to carry another baby for us. We think, also, about Catherine's future. We plan to introduce her to the concept of surrogate motherhood at an early age, so that she will grow up familiar with the idea. We realize that ours is an unusual situation, and that challenges await us, but we think that our comfort with this process is ultimately what matters. Catherine will always know how much we wanted her.

9

The New Reproductive Technologies

T HE birth of Louise Brown in England in 1978 brought new hope to countless infertile couples. For the first time, women with absent or blocked tubes had the possibility of bearing children. Baby Louise was living proof that an egg fertilized outside the body—in vitro—could be reimplanted and result in a normal pregnancy.

In the decade since Louise Brown's birth, thousands of infertile couples have turned to IVF (in vitro fertilization) and, more recently, to GIFT (gamete intra fallopian transfer) as their last hope for biological parenthood. For many, this hope has turned to disappointment since the success rates, even in the best programs, are poor. There is about a 15 percent "take home baby" rate for IVF. GIFT may be slightly higher; current research is equivocal. For other couples, however, IVF and GIFT have brought the answer to their prayers. By October 1987, over three thousand children worldwide were conceived by these new reproductive technologies. And, as these procedures are becoming more commonplace, infertility specialists are using them more and more frequently to treat a wide array of infertility problems.

What are IVF and GIFT, and who can they help? For those who have not had personal experiences with them, the names conjure up an array of high-tech, science fiction-like images. In reality, these procedures are medical ordeals, designed to treat certain problems that cause infertility. In IVF, eggs extracted from the woman are fertilized in a test tube with the husband's sperm. After several cell divisions (approximately forty-eight hours after fertilization takes place), the embryos are reimplanted in the uterus, in the hope that one (or more) will attach to the lining and continue to grow. Since IVF bypasses a woman's tubes, it is particularly useful for women who have blocked or absent tubes. To varying degrees, it is also used to treat other kinds of infertility problems.

In GIFT, the extracted eggs are mixed with semen from the husband, and immediately put into the fallopian tube. If all goes well, one or more eggs will be fertilized and implanted in the uterus. GIFT is available only to couples when the woman has at least one potent tube. It is a recommended treatment for unexplained infertility and for some cases of male infertility. Both IVF and GIFT have been used with varying success in women who have endometriosis or cervical mucus problems.

Both IVF and GIFT begin with the woman taking substantial amounts of hormone medication over the course of several days, designed to stimulate follicular (egg) development. During this time, her estrogen levels are carefully monitored by daily blood tests and the maturing follicles are measured by ultrasound. Should the estrogen levels rise too slowly, or the follicles grow too rapidly, there is a good chance that she will be "canceled" for that cycle. In fact, a large percentage of those undergoing IVF are canceled during the course of a given cycle. Consequently, completing the cycle becomes the first goal.

If all goes well with the developing follicles, the next step is egg retrieval. Eggs can be retrieved by laparoscopy, or vaginally, by using ultrasound guided aspiration, the latter procedure having the advantage of not requiring general anesthesia. Whether the egg and sperm mixture is placed immediately in the tube (GIFT), or two days later in the uterus (IVF), the couple spends the second half of the cycle in suspense, waiting and wondering.

For those couples fortunate enough not to be canceled along the way, those final days of the cycle are exceptionally difficult. IVF patients who know they are carrying one or more embryos, have the sense that they are tentatively pregnant. They fear spontaneous abortion. For GIFT patients, there is more uncertainty—they do not even know if fertilization took place. For both groups, the outcome of the treatment is determined by an early pregnancy test, ten days to two weeks after ovulation.

The news that IVF or GIFT has failed is devastating. Not only must the couple mourn the loss of their longed-for unborn child, but they must also deal with the loss of the physical, emotional, and financial resources that have been spent for nothing. In addition to the enormous loss they face, the medical staff who once showered them with attention and support, are not generally available to help with what may be a lengthy grieving process.

Those couples whose pregnancy test is positive initially experience a short-lived period of ecstasy. The next phase of their life is extemely stressful. Now that the pregnancy is official, they are even more fearful of pregnancy loss. Conditioned to failure, those couples who have been successful, wait for something to go wrong. Well versed in statistics, they know that the chance of miscarriage is substantial. Couples with GIFT pregnancies have the added concern that the pregnancy may be ectopic.

Couples do not decide casually to attempt IVF or GIFT. Not only are the procedures themselves extremely stressful, but also the decision-making process that leads up to it can be painful and conflict-ridden for the couple. The latter must ask themselves many questions that involve a series of challenges. We will discuss each of them.

1. *Should we try IVF or GIFT, or one of the more conventional treatments?* IVF currently offers the only hope for women with irreversively blocked or absent tubes who wish to conceive a biological child. For couples with unexplained infertility, or with other diagnoses, the decision can be difficult. The new reproductive technologies are promising, but they are also stressful and expensive ordeals that involve certain medical risks. Usually, physicians recommend IVF or GIFT when all other options have proved fruitless, and if the woman is not too old. Statistics have shown that as women approach forty, the odds of IVF or GIFT working are slim.

2. *Which should we try—IVF or GIFT?* Couples with unexplained infertility or problems other than blocked fallopian tubes, have a choice between IVF or GIFT. Both procedures have advantages and disadvantages. At present, GIFT is usually a more invasive procedure, as it involves the use of general anesthesia. But it is quicker and somewhat less costly than IVF. IVF is primarily done by using ultrasound guided aspiration, either through the vagina or the bladder. Only local anesthesia is required. IVF is a longer, and thus more expensive technology, as the woman must wait two days after her eggs have been retrieved in order for the fertilized embryos to undergo the required number of cell divisions. The fertilized eggs must then be reimplanted. Thus it is a two-step process. Another advantage of IVF, in addition to requiring only local anesthesia, is that it indicates whether the sperm can fertilize the egg. Some clinics will only attempt GIFT after at least one attempt of IVF, or after a sperm penetration assay, so they can be sure that fertilization will occur. GIFT, as mentioned before, is faster and cheaper, and often preferred by patients. Eventually GIFT, too, will probably be done using ultrasound guided aspiration making it the treatment of choice, rather than IVF, for many infertility conditions. Unfortunately,

however, GIFT may carry with it a somewhat greater risk of an ectopic pregnancy.

3. *Should we try IVF or GIFT or donor insemination?* The new reproductive technologies are often used to treat male infertility problems, specifically low sperm count or poor motility. Many couples, however, decide to do donor insemination instead. Couples in this situation face a difficult dilemma. They would prefer a child that is biologically linked to both of them, but the emotional, physical, and financial cost involved in the new reproductive technologies is enormous, and usually unrewarding. If there are no known female factors, donor insemination offers them the likelihood of a pregnancy and a child that is genetically linked to one of them, without the difficulties involved in IVF or GIFT. Of course, there are other "costs" of using donor insemination (see chapter 8, "Half Biologically Ours: Donor Insemination and Surrogate Parenting") and because of them many couples choose the new reproductive technologies.

4. *Should we attempt one of the new reproductive technologies or adopt a child?* Most couples do not have unlimited financial resources. The new reproductive technologies are expensive and offer no assurance of a baby. In fact, the likelihood of a baby via one of these methods is fairly slim. Adoption, though it can be expensive (usually between eight and twenty thousand dollars depending on the type of adoption), almost always guarantees a baby if the couple successfully completes the homestudy. In some states, where private adoption is legal, a formal homestudy is not even required. Couples must decide how to best allocate their financial resources. They must answer several questions, such as, do they want to gamble on IVF or GIFT in the hope of getting their first choice—a biological baby? Or, are they willing to settle for their second choice route to getting a baby—adoption? Can they afford to try IVF and if it does not work, adopt? In answering these questions, couples must not only consider their financial resources, but they must also consider the physical and emotional resources they have for coping with the stress of IVF or GIFT.

5. *Having decided to try one of the new reproductive technologies, to which program do we apply?* Deciding on where to get treatment can be a difficult and confusing matter. Programs vary in their protocols and in their results. They vary in the ways in which they report their success rates. Real differences do exist and couples must look carefully at the way in which the different programs report their statistics. Are success rates measured by the percentage of positive pregnancy tests registered ten days to two weeks after the procedure is performed? Or, is the success rate determined by the number of preg-

nancies that result in live births? Couples sometimes decide to travel out of state to programs that are more promising than local ones. Since couples are spending an enormous amount of emotional and physical energy, as well as money, it is important that they maximize their chances for pregnancy.

6. *When, and for how many cycles, should we try IVF or GIFT?* As new technologies, IVF and GIFT get perfected each year. If age is not a factor, couples have the option to wait a few years until the techniques are improved. In the meantime, they may choose to adopt, or pursue other options. Older couples, in which the woman is approaching forty, should probably elect to have the procedure performed as soon as possible, should they choose IVF or GIFT.

Once a couple has attempted IVF or GIFT the question is how many subsequent attempts they should make, if the first one is not successful. For those without insurance coverage, finances may dictate when to stop. For those who have had a hard time physically or emotionally, the decision, again, may be easy. But those couples who can handle additional cycles may not know when to stop. Programs often recommend three or four attempts before stopping, but ultimately this difficult decision rests with the couple. Some need to go beyond four times in order to feel that they have done what they can; others find their emotional, financial, or physical resources "spent" much earlier.

7. *Should we try IVF or GIFT because they are available to us or can we say enough is enough?* This last question is, in many ways, the most difficult. There are some couples for whom the new reproductive technologies are more of a burden than a blessing. Some are frightened by the medications or the surgery that IVF and GIFT require; others may simply feel reluctant to spend so much time or money on something that offers so little promise of a return. But because they exist, IVF and GIFT are difficult to turn down. Infertile couples, for the most part, feel a need to try all avenues that are available.

In working with infertile couples considering these new technologies, we encourage them to look carefully at the questions that we have just outlined. Those who do go on to try one of them need support during the procedure, as well as afterwards, whatever the outcome. And those who decide to say no, also need support and understanding from helping professionals. They may feel particularly lonely, guilty, or even selfish. But they need to know that their decision was equally courageous.

We have chosen to supplement this chapter with Dawne Era's "An In Vitro Journey," an edited version, due to space limitations, of the journal she kept during her in vitro experience. Her journey takes the reader through the world of high technology, where love-making and conception cannot be further apart, where hopes are born . . . and lost. Her journal illustrates the sheer will and determination it takes to survive the month-long physical and emotional ordeal that will either end in joy or, unfortunately most often, in heartache.

An In Vitro Journey

Dawne Era

In order to go through in vitro fertilization in September, my period needed to fall between September 20th and 30th, due to the in vitro program's scheduling. We thought that would probably happen, as my August cycle started on the 24th. We just made it—I started to menstruate on the 21st. I decided to keep an account of our journey.

Day 1: Monday

We're calling today Day 1, even though I started spotting yesterday. We ran a five-mile road race yesterday at the hospital where Ed is a staff physician—afterwards I noticed the spotting. My first thought was that I wouldn't be running again for at least a month. The hardest part of this process is that I have to remain physically inactive—I am not a sedentary person, and one needs to be exactly that during an IVF cycle. Somehow, though, it doesn't feel as depressing this time as it did the last time. At least we will be actively doing something about getting a child, and maybe—no definitely—it will take our minds off the adoption that fell through last week. And I know what to expect—injections that never seem to end, daily blood drawing, ultrasounds, surgery. It won't be fun, but at least we still have the hope of having a biological child.

I canceled my appointments for this morning after I noticed the spotting yesterday. I got up at 6:00 A.M. to make the seventy minute drive to the hospital for a baseline ultrasound. I prayed on the way that there would be no follicles left over from last month, and all would be set to go. I worried about the fact that I still wasn't bleeding heavily: "What if it isn't really my period, but midcycle spotting and my period will be very late this cycle?" What else can I worry about?

The ultrasound—I waited pacing, sitting, going to the bathroom. I relieved my full bladder a tiny bit at a time for the half hour before I was called, only to discover that my bladder was too full! After emptying it somewhat, I lay back on the table more comfortably. The technician couldn't find my right ovary. My bowel was apparent, but not the ovary. My thoughts ranged from wondering whether she is new at doing ultrasounds, to imagining that my bowel had adhered to the ovary in the eleven months since our last IVF attempt. But the missing ovary finally appeared on the screen and I gave up on that fear. The ultrasound looked good—no follicles.

I took the report up to the IVF office and announced that my cycle had started. I was given instructions to begin Pergonal injections at 8:00 P.M. tomorrow, to be followed by injections each evening through Day 5. On Day 6, I am to report back to the hospital for ultrasound and blood tests.

Day 2: Tuesday

Ed and I were on a TV show today, as a representative infertile couple. I kept thinking, "It's really started, I ll get my first shot at 8:00 tonight." Going through this process makes being infertile very real. Other people make babies simply by making love.

Day 3: Wednesday

I worked today as usual—told my clients that I may need to cancel appointments on their day next week because I might be undergoing a medical procedure. As of now, there is no way of knowing what day next week it will be. I got my second shot tonight.

Day 5: Friday

I was aware of my ovaries working today—both feel enlarged a bit and active. Something is happening. I hope the ultrasound tomorrow shows enough follicles and that they are growing at the same rate so we won't be dropped from this cycle. Good news when I called the hospital today—tomorrow's ultrasound will be done using the vaginal probe—I won't have to go in with a full bladder again! I am doing better at getting the shots this time. I didn't even flinch tonight when Ed gave it to me. We are rotating—left arm, right arm, right buttock, left buttock, and then over again so I won't get too sore in any one spot. I still do not like the buttock shots, but at least I'm not crying this time—it's easier on Ed too.

Day 6: Saturday

Ed took a tube of blood from my arm before I got out of bed, so I wouldn't have to wait at the hospital to have it done. We left the house at 7:15 to arrive at the hospital in time for the 8:30 ultrasound appointment. I prayed during the drive that the follicles will be there in good number and even growth. I couldn't stand it, even at this point, if we had to stop now. The only positive would be that I could start running again. I really miss running—and sex and being able to have wine with dinner.

The vaginal probe ultrasound—what a breakthrough—no discomfort (or much less). My ovaries felt a little sore, but not having a full bladder made a tremendous difference. Good news today! Both ovaries are full of follicles of the appropriate size for Day 6. Relief! We can continue.

Day 7: Sunday

After having the ultrasound and dropping my blood off at the lab, we went to the IVF office so I could write out all the necessary checks. They totalled about $4,500. This elusive baby of ours has already cost us over $15,000 (for the medical treatments I've received and the IVF attempts).

I met with the anesthesiologist before leaving the hospital. Instead of general anesthesia, I will this time be having epidural anesthesia and remain awake during the egg retrieval. They have only recently begun using this method of retrieval. It eliminates the risks of general anesthesia, but I'm not wild about the thought of being awake.

When I called the hospital at 3:00 this afternoon, they confirmed that the egg retrieval will take place on Wednesday at 11:00 A.M. I am to get my HCG shot at 12:30 A.M. tonight. My estrogen level did almost double today. It's now 2250. I hope it doesn't double again—maybe that is not possible after the HCG. I don't know. We've set the alarm for 12:30; we're both too tired to stay awake.

Day 9: Tuesday

It's hard to believe that this cycle started only one week ago—it seems at least a month. It has taken over every aspect of my life. It is even difficult to walk at this point because my ovaries are so heavy. Ed had to give me two shots at 12:30 last night because the volume wouldn't fit into the size needles we have.

I started obsessing about the possibility of ovulating early, after I was told by one of the other women going through an IVF attempt this month that someone in the last cycle had ovulated before surgery. I can't imagine what that would be like. I'm also concerned about the procedure tomorrow. I know there is risk with any surgery, and signing the papers with the anesthesiologist yesterday made me start thinking about it. I don't want to die trying to get pregnant. All day long, I have tried to tell myself, "Of course that won't happen. You're being silly."

I put in a long day at work—didn't get home until 9:00 P.M. Ed and I ate dinner—I have to remember not to eat or drink between now and tomorrow at 11:00. That shouldn't be hard to do, as the surgery is all I'm thinking about.

Day 11: Thursday

I made it through! So much for all the comments I've heard about transvaginal being a breeze, though. At least I didn't get nauseous; the last time I was still vomiting the day after. The IV went in easier this time—I used relaxation and didn't even flinch. But the epidural was another story—it did hurt. The procedure took about an hour and a half. The worst part was afterwards when the epidural wore off in the recovery room. I had such tremendous back pain (probably from the position that I was in during the surgery) that I needed to get a shot of painkiller. I slept in the back seat on the drive home.

We should hear from the embryologist this afternoon and find out whether the eggs fertilized. They retrieved twelve or thirteen, as I remember, but will probably only fertilize six because they will put all the fertilized eggs into my uterus. Maybe I can catch up on some reading and writing during these next four days in bed.

Day 12: Friday

We had to be at the hospital early today for the embryo transfer. We spoke to the embryologist yesterday afternoon and found out that four eggs had fertilized. I was instructed to take Valium upon arrival at the hospital. The transfer was easy—no pain—I just wish we could have seen the embryos before they were put in. After the transfer, I stayed on my back in the recovery room for four hours and was then wheeled out. I laid in the back seat of the car and slept most of the way home and most of the afternoon and evening. I'm still tired.

I am visualizing the embryos trying to attach to the uterine wall. Please let it work this time, God. We have waited so long and tried so hard. We want this baby so much! We are not the only ones invested in this baby. Our daughter (my biological daughter from an earlier marriage, Ed's step-daughter), who is nineteen and a sophomore in college, has also been waiting five years for us to have this baby. Even though she is living away from home now, the two adoptions that fell through and the failed IVF attempt were hard for her, too. And it's been hard for Ed's parents and my mother and all our siblings who are waiting to be aunts and uncles to our baby. We deserve this baby—we know we will be good parents. Infertility has taken its toll on us. It seems as if it has been forever. I have to be hopeful, but I am so tired.

Day 13: Saturday

I became very depressed this afternoon. I wonder whether it's the proges-terone shot I got last night. Only thirteen more to go. They are the most painful shots I've ever had. I'm sure to be very sore in all four shot spots by the end of this, and if I get pregnant (*please God*) I will continue to get the shots for another fourteen days. I probably won't care at all then. It seems like two months since this cycle started, and I'm very low—physically, men-tally, spiritually. I do feel a bit sexual for the first time in two weeks, but that's out for at least two more weeks, and if I get pregnant, it's out for three more months. Seems a small price to pay after all these years and treatments.

I'm suddenly pessimistic about the possibility of becoming pregnant. All the feelings of the last failed cycle came back today, and I mentally went through the two cycles comparing each part of the process—what was alike and what was different, and with each difference, trying to conjure up hope within myself that this time it will happen. I also had flashes of conversations I've had with people recently. Two close friends have said they have a good feeling. When I told this to Ed a couple of days ago, he mentioned that a friend of ours said that the last time, too. I know he wants to keep our hopes tempered so the devastation, if I don't get pregnant, will not be so bad. I know it will be bad anyway. This is truly too much to go through not to get pregnant. The prospect is too bleak. I'm so depressed. . . . I need to muster up some hope soon.

Day 14: Sunday

I slept restlessly throughout the night—got up three times to urinate—had pain in my abdomen. Ed's first words this morning were, "You can get up to-day." I did so for the first time, careful not to jostle my body in any way—still concerned about the embryos falling out. Ed went to church this morning to pray for us. I stayed home and visualized the embryos attaching to my womb. Implantation takes place sometime around Day 5 after the transfer. I'm trying to give them a good start.

Day 23: Tuesday

I haven't written for over a week. It seems like a month has gone by. I had a pregnancy test done today, even though we are supposed to wait until Day 26. Ed said it should show up by now. I waited for Ed to call me at work with the results, as the lab was to call his office. I fantasized all day that he would call me and excitedly say, "It's positive!" But instead when he called, I heard him say that we'd wait until Friday and have another test—there's still a chance. I began to feel very unpregnant in my progesterone stimulated body. My breasts are enlarged, and physically I look and feel like an impregnated woman. At least my body doesn't look and feel the way it usually does. It's hard to believe that it's just the progesterone.

Oh God, please don't let this happen to us again. In the five years of our marriage, we have lost our baby again and again. Each time my period started—sixty times. How many more losses can we take? It can't be; we thought everything went well this time. What happened to our embryos? I have become so attached to them.

Day 24: Wednesday

I started spotting this afternoon. I called Ed. He was surprised that my period would override the progesterone. I know we were both thinking that maybe, just maybe, the spotting was from the embryo implanting. But it's too late for that kind of bleeding—that should have happened seven days ago. I can't believe we're going through this again.

I cried when Ed gave me my progesterone shot tonight—in case all the indications are wrong and I am pregnant. We are just waiting for Friday to come. Right now, I just want this to be over.

Day 26: Friday

My period became heavy this morning, but I went to have the pregnancy test anyway. After all, pregnant women can have bleeding. Since Tuesday, despite all the indications that I am not pregnant, we have held out hope for a miracle—that the pregnancy test results would be positive today. I felt abused as the blood was drawn from my arm. I also felt a morbid amusement that I was even there getting a pregnancy test.

Ed got the results this afternoon and called me. "No surprises." I am feeling numb right now. We kept this night free and made a reservation at a nice restaurant so that we could celebrate the good news or soothe ourselves in the event of bad news. We canceled our reservation because neither of us felt like going to a place we reserve for good times. This is truly a bad time.

10
Secondary Infertility

T HE inability to conceive, or carry to term, a second pregnancy, after a woman has already given birth to one child, is termed secondary infertility. Couples who experienced infertility prior to the birth of a first child expect to be infertile again. However, for couples who had little or no difficulty conceiving their first child, secondary infertility comes as a shock. Because a couple once conceived with ease, they are often more surprised about their condition than are couples who are facing infertility for the first time.

Couples with secondary infertility experience many of the same feelings, conflicts, and difficulties that accompany primary infertility. They get angry at themselves and at the world. They often feel inadequate psychologically as well as physically. They may feel empty and incomplete, despite the fact that they do have a child. In addition, they feel isolated—different from fertile families, but also very different from the majority of infertile couples who have primary infertility. Those who have not been able to conceive at all envy those who have had a child. The concept of secondary infertility seems foreign to men and women who may be silently bargaining with the spiritual world for the birth of just one healthy baby.

Frequently, the grief of couples with secondary infertility is not recognized or acknowledged by friends or family. Having a child is a ticket to parenthood. Music lessons, car pools, or PTA meetings camouflage the suffering of couples who are desperate for another child. Even friends who know that a couple would like more children have no idea of the despair the latter may feel. After all, others might reason, they should be grateful for the one child they have. Couples with secondary infertility are grateful for their child, but they are painfully aware of what they do not have—more children to complete their families.

Most couples, at some point in their relationship, set goals for themselves in relation to work and family. They dream and they plan. Couples who choose to have more than one child and discover they are infertile, experience an interruption of their life plan. They feel incomplete and unfulfilled. Sometimes these couples own large homes with several bedrooms, purchased with the expectation of filling them up. Family portraits look empty; their home is too quiet. To compound their sadness, innocent others often ask the dreaded question, "When are you going to have another child?"

Couples with secondary infertility are often puzzled about their situation. It may feel like an assault on their bodies and a blow to their self-esteem. In an attempt to attach meaning to this unexpected fate, many couples blame themselves. Sometimes they feel they are being punished for over-indulging—perhaps by excessive eating, drinking, or using drugs. Others may feel guilty about an affair or an indiscretion. Most common of all is the fear that their secondary infertility is a confirmation of the sad truth—that they are not good enough parents. That feeling of being inadequate as a parent is usually the most difficult emotion to face, and can lead to a diminished ability to receive pleasure from the child they have already borne.

Most parents contemplating a second child worry that he or she will not be as special or as wonderful as their first. They may wonder how they could possibly feel as attached to number two, convinced that no child—not even one they produce—could come close to their first offspring. They fear the unspeakable—that they just won't love another child as much as they love their first. Thus couples with secondary infertility, in addition to blaming themselves for being inadequate parents, often blame themselves for their ambivalence as well. They forget that hesitations or doubts about a second child are normal.

Parents who want more than one child think about the ideal spacing of their children. Most couples prefer that their children not be too far apart in years. As they watch their only child getting older, they realize that their fantasies of closeness are beyond their grasp. They alter their plans and fervently hope for another child, even if his or her birth is far removed from their first.

Couples unable to have another child often become terrified that their only child will die. They fear cancer and they fear cars. In a desperate attempt to avoid their nightmare, they may cling even more tenaciously to their child. They try not to smother, but feel an added need to protect. Their infertility has made them more vulnerable to loss.

Couples with secondary infertility, like couples with primary infertility, must put their lives on hold for a while. Plans to move, plans to change careers, or plans to go back to school, often get pushed in the background while couples are consumed with temperature charts and doctor's visits. Many women plan to return to work when their children reach a certain age. Though many women with secondary infertility may desire to work, they may be reluctant to get too involved in a career they might have to give up, should they be lucky enough to conceive. When their child reaches pre-school or school age, their identity, as well as their self-esteem, suffers. With no job and no baby at home for whom to care, they may feel stuck in their life, lacking purpose or meaning.

Thus the feelings of loss experienced by couples with secondary infertility, are tinged with guilt, fear, and feelings of inadequacy. Most of these feelings are not recognized or understood by others, often not even by helping professionals. Yet the loss is enormous for those who are in the midst of it.

In working with couples with secondary infertility, we stress that their situation is a particularly lonely one, acknowledging that they do not feel like they belong in either the fertile or the infertile world. We encourage them to find others in the same position. Local RESOLVE chapters are usually a good resource. We try to help them weigh alternatives to their infertility—adoption or having just one child—if a medical solution cannot be found. Though we empathize with their plight and help them express their feelings of loss, we also point out the advantages of having children who are spaced far apart, whether it be by birth or adoption, as well as the advantages of having one child. In "Just As Bad This Time," Vivian Finkelstein captures the frustration and anguish of those who have one child and long for another.

Just As Bad This Time

Vivian Finkelstein

I know that infertility hurts, whether it's primary or secondary, because I had both. I thought that the second time would be easier because I was prepared for it. I was wrong.

After two years of secondary infertility, I decided to try Pergonal as a last resort. I became pregnant on the fourth cycle, but I had an early miscarriage. After a two-month break, I became pregnant on the next Pergonal cycle, but miscarried again. The first miscarriage left my husband and me feeling optimistic because I had finally conceived again. But the second one left us feeling uncertain and less hopeful. I was afraid to try again, but did not want to give up either. We took a long summer break, then I resumed Pergonal and became pregnant on the second cycle. After a difficult pregnancy, which included spotting, loss of a twin, cerclage surgery, and a great deal of anxiety, I gave birth to a healthy baby girl in July 1986.

Many of my feelings while undergoing treatment for secondary infertility were the same as those I experienced with primary infertility. The fact that I already had a child didn't make me feel any better. I still felt like a failure and wondered how I would get through the days, weeks, and months ahead. This time, unlike the first, I faced the expense and anxiety of Pergonal, and the ultrasounds that I hated more than the shots. The belief that I had nothing to look forward to but more of the same, was depressing. I felt just as devastated the second time around, when I got my period. My body was failing me, and the fact that it had once succeeded was no comfort.

I also felt the same feelings of jealousy and depression when I learned of other women's pregnancies and births, and saw their babies. I could be happy for someone having her first child, but not her second. What made it more difficult was that I couldn't avoid being around mothers with two children, unless I wanted to deprive my daughter of a normal childhood. My daughter was in a playgroup, and two of the women had babies according to their schedules, while I had to undergo tests, shots, and ultrasounds month after month.

Nursery school was also very painful. All I focused on were pregnant moms, or moms with babies or toddlers waiting outside the door. By the time Marla was four years old, we seemed to be constantly surrounded by mothers with at least two children. I often endured the question, "Is she your only child?" At kindergarten orientation we were asked if she was our first or last child starting school. I sat there wondering if it had ever occurred to anyone that Marla could be our first *and* last child.

I had the same feeling of life being put on hold, as I did the first time I was trying to conceive. Should I look for a job, or wait, hoping that soon I would be pregnant? How long should we continue treatment? Should we seriously consider adoption? Should we take our vacation and miss two precious cycles?

The second time, I had additional questions to consider. I wondered if I should give away my maternity clothes. Maybe it was bad luck keeping them around; it certainly was depressing. Should I finally put the high chair and changing table in the basement? Everything was in limbo, just as before, until we would either succeed or give up our struggle. I played the same mind game with clothing as I had before, hating to buy something because I might be pregnant the next month and it wouldn't fit. I again used the chance of a pregnancy as an excuse for not living in the present.

I kept wondering why this was happening to us. Although I asked this question often the first time, my feelings were even stronger the second time. Why was I being punished twice? It was supposed to be easier, now that I thought I knew what my problems were. I had never had a miscarriage before; now I had had two. I had not taken Pergonal the first time. My pregnancy with Marla had been uneventful. To undergo infertility treatment once, and then have to struggle with additional complications the second time, seemed most unfair.

With secondary infertility, I knew what I was missing. The first time all I knew was that I wanted a baby. This time, I wanted so badly to experience being pregnant again—to feel the baby kick, to watch it being born, and especially to nurse. I had tasted chocolate and I wanted it again.

Perhaps the most difficult aspect of secondary infertility, was the feeling of not belonging to either the fertile or infertile world. I felt like a misfit. I felt guilty for even mentioning that I had a child when I attended RESOLVE meetings. I guessed that childless couples would not understand what I had to complain about, and would resent my being there. I felt that I had to apologize for being a mother, which was an awful feeling, because I too had struggled with primary infertility. I really wanted to share my story with others because I did not have any support when I was trying to become pregnant with Marla. My RESOLVE chapter did not exist then, and infertility was not openly discussed the way it is now. But when I went to get help the second time around, I found I had been correct in my prediction. Others did not understand that I was also feeling depressed, angry, and frustrated, even though I had a child.

Back in the fertile world I had to listen to comments such as, "Raising two kids is so much more work; be glad you only have one." Or, "After all you went through, be grateful you have a child at all. Some women can't have any." Of course, those who made these comments had two or more children, and their pregnancies were planned according to the seasons in which they wanted to be pregnant. Sometimes they would say things like, "Oh, she's an only child. That's why she is so dependent on you." It was difficult enough to cope with being almost the only parent in nursery school, playgroup, ballet, or kindergarten with only one child. It was worse feeling chastized because of it.

No one seemed to understand how I was feeling, except those with secondary infertility. With them I could be proud of my daughter, but I could also share feelings of sadness, anger, and frustration. It was difficult to find others with secondary infertility, but it was such a relief when I did. I participated in a RESOLVE support group just for women with this problem. We were so glad to have found each other that some of us decided to continue meeting after the formal support group ended. We included our children so that they could play while we talked. Eventually more women joined the network and meetings were changed to the evening so that we could discuss issues more freely without the children being present. The formal support group and the informal network helped me to understand and cope with my infertility. There will always be a special bond among those of us who shared our feelings during that period. I was also grateful for the support I received during my difficult and very risky pregnancy.

The effect of infertility on our daughter was, of course, a concern to my husband and me. We never made up excuses about my doctor's visits. Marla knew that we were trying to have another baby. We kept the explanation simple: we wanted her to have a brother or a sister, but it was not happening, so we needed the doctor to help us. Often she asked to come with me to doctor's appointments, and I was glad to have her company. I don't know what she will remember as an adult, but she knows now that couples don't always have babies when they choose, and that it can be a long and painful process.

Marla's reaction to the baby was more positive than I had anticipated. She was thrilled to have a sister! After more than six years of our complete attention, I thought she would be more jealous, but that stage lasted only a few weeks. Perhaps the adjustment has been so easy because the age difference between them lessens the competition. I would never have chosen such a large age span, but it does have its advantages. Marla was busy with first grade activities when Pamela was born. She was not with her all day, so when she came home from school, she would always kiss and hug her. She kept asking me when she could bring her for Show and Tell. Because we included her in the infertility process, she realizes how special Pammie is, and how grateful we are finally to be a family of four!

11

Moving On
or:
When Is Enough, Enough?

W HEN is enough, enough? Couples experiencing long-term infertility
ask themselves this question often, yet most couples find that asking the question is much simpler than arriving at the answer. Rapid advances
in the treatment of infertility make it increasingly difficult to say that a situation is hopeless, and physicians are seemingly reluctant to suggest that infertile couples give up and move on. Without a clearly designated signpost that
says "end of the road," couples are left to determine for themselves, when
they can go no further.

For some couples, the decision to quit is fairly straightforward. Some suffer from problems for which treatment is either unavailable or perhaps offers
minimal hope. Others share an aversion to medical tests and treatment and
are prepared to adopt or live childfree rather than subject themselves to more
experiences that they anticipate will be frightening, painful, intrusive, and
very possibly disappointing.

Most infertile couples do not quit easily. Most prize the opportunity to
have a child, and willingly enter into the long process of tests and treatments.
Many feel that they must try all avenues before they can consider giving up.
Some assume that if there were really no hope their physician would say so.
They reason that as long as further treatments are offered, then they must be
advisable.

So couples move along trying one treatment, then another. Depending on
their diagnosis, there are a range of approaches that can be tried. Finances
and fortitude play a part in determining how many times any one technique
or treatment is attempted. But sooner or later, one spouse or the other
declares, "I've had it, I cannot go on, enough is enough." Often this is the

partner who has undergone the bulk of tests and treatment while her (it usually is a "her") spouse has been much less involved.

For some couples, the announcement by one member, that enough is enough, precipitates a crisis. Often the other partner, though perhaps more passive, is by no means interested in giving up. In fact, he or she may just be gearing up for more involvement. The first partner may find some renewed strength from a declaration of participation, or may hold fast to the position that enough really is enough. Other couples encounter a different dilemma: they may agree that they are approaching the end of the line, but disagree on a second choice. Debates about adoption versus donor insemination versus childfree living, keep them locked in unproductive treatment regimens.

Finally, there are couples in which either one or both partners ascribe to the "leave not a stone unturned" philosophy. These are individuals who do not give up as long as there is a treatment that they have not tried, or an opportunity to try a familiar treatment one last time. In fact, some physicians keep providing encouragement to continue trying, which only contributes to their patients' dilemma. Occasionally, physicians advise their patients to move on and consider other options, when they believe that further treatment would be fruitless.

In working with infertile couples, we try to be tolerant of variations in pace and energy. We feel that people need to be reminded that there is no right or wrong way to be infertile; couples must simply decide what is best for them. There is no shame attached to "quitting," and there may be no rewards for heroism. But couples must also know that to give up before they both feel ready to do so is likely to delay resolution. For it is difficult to wholeheartedly pursue other alternatives if they are still wondering whether they should have had surgery or tried yet another medication.

With rapid advances in reproductive medicine, some couples have the option of deciding that enough is enough, knowing that they may later change their minds and resume treatment. Those whose age and diagnosis make this possible, may need help acknowledging that it is reasonable to temporarily stop treatment. Should they interrupt treatment they then face additional questions regarding adoption, and possibly either donor insemination or surrogate mothering. It is certainly a complex matter to move on to any of these "second choices" when their first choice remains a possibility.

In helping infertile couples decide when enough is enough, we suggest that they consider six questions. The answers to these questions should help couples clarify the issues involved and arrive at a decision:

1. How important is it to us to have a biological child versus no child, or an adopted child?

2. How much longer can we tolerate the uncertainty of whether we will conceive a child?

3. How much more physical pain and risk can we take?

4. Are we willing to continue to have our daily routine interrupted by necessary medical tests and regimens?

5. To what extent has our relationship been negatively affected by infertility?

6. Can we afford (and do we choose) to spend more money on potentially expensive treatments?

1. *How important is it for us to have a biological child (versus adopting or having no child)?* This question is often the most difficult. Couples must come to terms with what it means to have or desire a biological child. Most people discover, sometimes surprisingly, that their ego is involved. It is the rare couple who have no interest in propagating his curly blond hair, her musical talent, or their "intelligent genes." Almost everyone has at least some stake in preserving a part of themselves for posterity.

For women, having a biological child also means experiencing pregnancy, childbirth, and nursing. From an early age, girls view childbearing as an essential life event—the reason for which their bodies were made. As we have said before, difficulty in conceiving or carrying a pregnancy has serious impact on the way a woman views herself and her body.

Thus, the inability to have a biological child involves two major losses: the inability to carry on one's genetic link and the inability to fulfill one's biological destiny. Each category of loss contains within it many smaller losses, and each couple must acknowledge what all the losses mean to them, both separately and as a couple. If they are not ready to begin this process, then perhaps they are not ready to end treatment.

2. *How much longer can we tolerate the uncertainty of not knowing if and when we will conceive?* In considering the second question, couples must think about what it means to spend the second half of each cycle on pins and needles. The week or two before menstruation is a very stressful time for women, who look for any signs and signals that might indicate pregnancy. Their husbands often become anxious sometimes as a response to their

wives' moods. Couples must decide how much longer they can tolerate these monthly cycles of anxiety, uncertainty, and despair. Stopping treatment can enable them to finally step off the roller coaster.

3. *How much more physical risk and pain can we take?* The diagnosis and treatment of infertility involves physical, as well as emotional, risk and pain. Our third question encourages couples to look at how much more one or both partners can undergo physically. With long-term infertility, some unpleasant tests, such as the endometrial biopsy and the hysterosalpingogram, may need to be repeated periodically. The laparoscopy, which requires general anesthesia, may also need to be repeated. Couples, and particularly women (since they often undergo the major physical interventions, even in situations of male infertility), must decide whether they can handle further physical risk and pain. If the answer is no, or doubt is increasing, it may be time to interrupt or terminate treatment.

4. *How many more disruptions can we tolerate?* Infertility specialists, like most professionals, work during the day. It is the patients who must disrupt their daily work schedules and make the necessary accommodations, in order for their infertility to be treated. Most individuals, men and women, find these accommodations to be an extreme hardship, no matter how desperately they may want a child. Surely, it is difficult to advance in one's job when much time is being taken off for "mysterious" reasons.

Careers suffer in other ways. Men and women, though more often the latter, often postpone career plans, anticipating a pregnancy. Couples nearing the end of the infertility road may feel that it is time to spend less time in doctor's offices and pharmacies and more time pursuing other areas of their lives.

5. *To what extent does infertility have a negative effect on our relationship and how long can that continue?* Infertility always adds stress to a marriage. Usually, a couple's sexual relationship is what suffers the most. After several months of scheduled sex, a couple has little desire to make love spontaneously. What was once a pleasurable act is now frought with so much pain that it feels better to avoid it altogether. The end result is often that a husband and wife feel more distant from each other, since a primary means of expressing intimacy is no longer available to them.

Infertility takes a chunk out of people's lives. It creates a developmental halt that is sometimes seen more easily in retrospect. In deciding whether enough is enough, couples must evaluate the damage done to their careers and to their relationship. They need to determine whether these major aspects of their lives can withstand more "time off."

6. *Can we afford to spend money on potentially expensive treatments?* The first five questions address issues of emotional stress, loss, or physical pain. This sixth question is purely financial. Health insurance providers do not ordinarily cover infertility treatment; they cover only patients whose diagnosis relates to certain medical conditions. Pergonal shots are extremely expensive. Artificial inseminations, both with husband and with donor sperm, can also be quite costly. So can many other tests and treatments for infertility. In vitro fertilization (IVF) and gamete intra fallopian transfer (GIFT) probably the most "high-tech" of the treatments, costs several thousand dollars per attempt, and the chances of success are only about 20 percent. Couples, at least those in relatively secure financial situations, are sometimes forced to decide whether to spend their savings on a new house or on four cycles of in vitro.

Adoption, though not a medical treatment, can also be quite expensive. Couples who are candidates for IVF or GIFT must decide whether to spend their money on adoption—a better bet, but their second choice, or on in vitro—lower odds, but a preferred outcome. These decisions are, of course, difficult. Couples must determine their priorities and decide how to spend their financial resources.

In helping couples decide when to stop treatment, it is important to understand that when the door is finally closed on treatment, it is not necessarily shut tightly. Probably all couples, even those who are reasonably certain of their decision, have regrets from time to time. They may wonder whether one more cycle of intrauterine insemination would have done the trick, or whether they should have risked the tubal surgery despite the very low odds. Unless infertility is conclusive, and it usually is not, some small amount of hope lingers. Deciding when to stop treatment and pursue other options is an important step toward resolution, but it does not mean that all hope is automatically extinguished. Advances in reproductive medicine make it possible for some couples who have 'given up" to decide to resume treatment if or when some new "hope" becomes available.

In the pages that follow are four essays written by women in the process of moving on after deciding that enough is enough. Teri Flinn presents a poignant account of her attempt to grieve a child who was never born, though very much desired. Lois Gillooly talks about her experience of moving on, from the perspective of someone who has had multiple miscarriages. Her resolution is adoption, which provides her with a new, though different, hope. Sally Chapralis offers a witty account of her experience with infertil-

ity, telling it with some hindsight, as well as awareness, of what the future
may or may not bring. Maggie Rogers, whose mother was nicknamed "Fertile Myrtle," chronicles her struggle with infertility and expresses the relief
she feels as she recognizes her own ability to move away from the pain and
on with her life. We end this chapter with "Mother's Day," in which
Margaret Munk poetically expresses the dilemma of deciding when enough
is enough.

Taps in the Cabbage Patch

Teri Flinn

It is November 11th and in the morning newspaper there's a photo of a
woman and her young son comforting each other. There is a folded flag
between them. They are attending a burial at Arlington cemetery. Their
tears are fresh but the body they are burying has been dead for thirteen
years. It is the body of a man missing in action in Vietnam. The obituary
lists his age at twenty-seven. I guess he's still twenty-seven, but I somehow
find that strange. I've often heard how important it is for families to have a
body to grieve over. Apparently, people cannot put closure on a relationship
till they go through the grieving process. The pain on their faces is not thirteen years old.

On television that same day, I hear that the Channel 4 reporter has just
died of head injuries he received in a crash last week. I see reruns of the
reporter's face as I saw it countless times before. I never noticed him that
much, but now I know all about him, his wife, and his little baby girl. I feel
the shock of his death as if it is my own. I am feeling dead. I wonder how his
wife will take this blow. Her husband and their future together are dead.

I can't get beyond the blow I took myself the day before. It was our fifth
year of infertility treatment here in Boston. We have one son who is growing up. He was conceived after several years of tests that only alluded to an
antibody problem with the sperm. I was having a routine test to determine
my exact time of ovulation and suddenly the pain was too great. When he
finished, the doctor seemed shaken. He said that my uterus had been scarred
by the Caesarean birth and that an infection had set in. I never had had a
chance at another conception. Five years of operations, tests, inseminations,
temperature charts, and drugs had been a complete waste of time and
money.

At first, I felt a sense of relief. Some reason had finally been found. I felt as if the life support systems to a dream had been shut off and there was blessed release in that. This hope had been held alive too long by artificial means. Then the reality set in. I called a counselor from RESOLVE, the support group for infertility patients. I told her I felt as if someone had died. She said that this was a good sign and that my problem for so long was that I could not mourn for this loss.

How could I mourn when there was no body? Each of those sixty months I could try desperately not to build up my hopes, but the secret thoughts would creep in and the baby names would filter through. Each month, the imaginary presence would dissolve in a pool of blood. It was a death only I saw and only I felt. There were no flowers for me, no condolence cards, no markers. I would see the more tangible evidence that life went on in other women as their babies were born and began to toddle and then to walk. I'd open the Christmas cards from friends and count two little heads where there once was one and then the next year count three. Some people knew of my sadness but they never talked of it. They'd talk about others' deaths and miscarriages, but who feels for the unformed life?

The counselor wants me to bring in an item of baby clothes to cry over. I won't do that. Not with a stranger. I had an idea long ago that I guess I will enact now. I will buy a Cabbage Patch Doll, the cutest one I can find. I've secretly wanted one, but my son won't even look at them. I will dress her in the little red and white outfit my baby wore home from the hospital. It was the only thing I had the courage to buy before he was born. It took a leap of faith to buy it and I loved the little red striped fish embroidered on it.

I will dress her carefully and kiss her goodbye. I will put her in a small box. She will be buried in my flower garden . . . and I will cry. I will do it alone because this has been my dream and my obsession. I pursued it no matter what the odds. My husband will not be there to see the tears. He has seen too many. My son will not see his sibling buried. It will be over and there will be no more months of hope.

But there will be days of living . . . living with life as it really is. Not as I wish it to be. I have never lost anyone close to me, and I now know how unprepared I am to face a loss. I could not believe there was something in life I could not do. I didn't think I'd ever let life stop me. Now I know that there are things that happen to us over which we have no control. You have to put an end to that sadness. You have to find the body and bury it. You have to grieve and then go on living.

The dark November clouds roll by the burial places—the soldier, the reporter, the Cabbage Patch kid. Dare I compare my grief with those women? I don't know. The random acts of life have forged their stories. The grieving and the healing begins.

It's Spring Again

Lois A. Gillooly

Bob and I had been trying to conceive for two years. I occasionally worried that there might be a problem. Then I'd talk myself out of it by blaming Bob's business trips for ruining the right timing. I did know that I was a DES daughter. At an annual exam conducted under a federally-funded DES study, after the first fruitless year, I asked if anything in my medical record might explain my delay in getting pregnant. I was told that there was no apparent problem, and that getting pregnant with two was better than trying with three—in other words, I was told to give it more time before consulting a doctor. While we waited, and while there were two incomes, we bought a larger house. A friend who had finally gotten pregnant after several years of trying, awarded me her basal thermometer, and introduced me to tempera-ture charts. I usually was able to believe that when the time was "right," it would happen. I just couldn't figure out why it wasn't "right" yet.

In the spring of 1984, the pregnancy test results were positive. We were elated. We calculated the due date. In fact, the due date would be exactly a year after two friends had surprised everyone by delivering their first babies on the same day. We made announcements to family and friends; we talked about names. Then suddenly, it was over. I was at the airport meeting my mother, who was returning from Texas after visiting my sister and her new baby. I didn't feel quite right. I had some cramping, just like my period cramping; and then the spotting started. I felt that something was terribly wrong. The doctor wasn't alarmed at the spotting. It didn't always mean trouble. I kept hoping against hope. But the pregnancy ended a few days later, when I had a spontaneous abortion at about day forty.

That first spring was still so hopeful. While I was terribly disappointed, I felt that some progress had been made, since I had gotten pregnant. Everyone made optimistic comments: "But at least you know you can get pregnant." "One in five pregnancies ends in miscarriage." "It's probably for the best. Something must have been wrong with the embryo." "Oh, don't worry. You'll be pregnant again soon." I wanted to believe everything that was said, and I did.

My expectation had been to have a baby before I was thirty-five. I was about to turn thirty-six. I felt there was no time to waste. We consulted an infertility specialist, and spent the next year trying to determine if there was a problem. I can remember the doctor telling Bob and me that the hospital had counselors available if we should ever need to call upon them. I felt somewhat amused, and just a bit insulted. We were here to identify some minor physical problem, which the doctor would fix. There would be no need for psychiatric help.

I learned to stick a thermometer in my mouth before I was fully awake each day. We had the usual run of tests and appointments that intruded on our most personal lives. One test showed two minor abnormalities, probably caused by my DES exposure: a slightly undersized womb and tubes that were thick at the bases. Neither condition was considered severe enough to be an identifiable cause of my difficulty getting pregnant, or my miscarriage.

In April and June of 1985, after a year of inconclusive testing, I had two, brief pregnancies that ended in miscarriage. I experienced a terrible roller coaster of emotion both times. My period would run late. ("I'm pregnant!") Then I would have some light staining at about day thirty-five. ("I'm not pregnant.") My temperature would remain elevated and the doctor would order tests. ("I'm pregnant!") Subsequent blood tests would show declining pregnancy hormone levels, and I would eventually miscarry. Now I had qualified for an ugly title—"Habitual Aborter." The medical question changed from "Why was I not getting pregnant?" to "Why was I miscarrying?"

In order to discover why I kept miscarrying, I was first tested for mycoplasma, an infection that is a cross between a virus and a bacteria. The test was positive. I was thrilled to be infected! Mycoplasma is suspected to be a cause of early miscarriage in some cases, and I believed that this would be the answer for me. The infection was treated, and for another year we continued with tests, treatments, and attempts to get pregnant.

So, in spite of the emotional costs of the second "pregnant" spring, there was some promise. There was an identified problem, which had been fixed, and the next time I got pregnant I wouldn't miscarry; I just wouldn't! I turned thirty-seven that July. The biological clock was ticking. It was beginning to be very difficult to see other women getting pregnant, often the very first month that they decided to try. Princess Di got pregnant; Jane Pauley got pregnant; everyone seemed to be pregnant except me. In my immediate family and close circle of friends, four babies were born that year.

As summer turned to fall, and fall to winter, Bob and I occasionally discussed the possibility of adoption. In November or December, when I had gotten my period once again and I was home from work on what I called a "mental health" day, I picked up the telephone book and called a few adoption agencies. The waiting period for the introductory or informational meetings was several months long, but I felt that I was doing something by getting on a few lists. Then, in February and March, we attended two informational meetings and a three-hour seminar on various types of adoption. The news was not great. Healthy, white infants were few and far between. Most agencies had waiting lists of five years and more. Having a biological child would be faster and more economical.

Then, in May of 1986, another spring, I had my fourth miscarriage. This time I felt no hope, and no promise. My doctor, who had a wonderful way of making me feel I was his only patient, was moving on to a new hospital. I was referred to another doctor who worked with women who had had multiple miscarriages. This doctor ordered more tests, but they were tests for things like lupus and chromosome abnormalities, conditions that caused only a small percentage of miscarriages. As the direction of the tests became more and more obscure, I began to feel like a laboratory experiment. I was nearing my thirty-eighth birthday. For the first time, I began to think that I might never bear a child. Confronting that possibility was the hardest thing I have ever had to face. It was the death of a dream.

Now all the comments from family and friends, meant to be comforting, had a hollow ring. "But at least you know you can get pregnant." (Sure, but then I miscarry!) "One in five pregnancies ends in miscarriage." (I'm no longer in the general population on which that statistic is based. My statistics are four for four.) "It's probably for the best." (But I want a child. Not having a child is not what I consider "for the best.") "Something must have been wrong with the embryo." (No. Something is wrong with me.) "Oh, don't worry. You'll be pregnant again soon." (In another year? And then another miscarriage? And I'll be thirty-nine.)

I began to cry. I cried often. I cried everywhere—at work, in bed, on the train. I distanced myself from nieces and nephews and the children of friends, born during the past two years. I played and interacted with the older children, but I couldn't pick up the infants. The smaller ones were the ages of the children I should have had.

I felt that there was no one in my life who could really understand how I felt. My family and friends all seemed to get pregnant by accident or in the very first month of trying. My husband had a biological child from an earlier marriage; and he actually felt guilty, he told me, that he did not have the depth of grief that I was experiencing.

At an adoption forum just after my last miscarriage, I had become aware of a medical consultant at RESOLVE, who would review your medical history with you, to identify any unexplored avenues of treatment. I really wanted to find out that we had explored all avenues, so that continued medical treatment would be ruled out and a biological child would no longer be an option. Then I would be forced to look at alternatives. Bob and I went for a consultation, but the answer I wanted wasn't presented to me in any neat little package. There were still more medical possibilities that could be tried. None offered a great deal of hope, or any guarantee of success, or even an acceptable time frame.

It was suggested that we join a support group. This time I was not "amused" or "a bit insulted," as I had been when help was offered at my first doctor's appointment. I was desperate, and I knew I had nothing to lose.

The first of our twelve weekly meetings was incredible to me. There were four other couples, real flesh and blood people, in the room and they could really understand, on a gut level, the pain and loss that was eating me up. I now knew people who wanted children as badly as I did and who, for various reasons, could not have them at the drop of a hat.

During those twelve weeks, Bob and I set for ourselves a goal of deciding if adoption was what we wanted to do. We had to separate out two parts of parenting: the physical giving of life and the lifelong raising of a child to adulthood. Did we still want to partake of the lifelong commitment, with the knowledge that the physical act of giving birth was not possible? Or did we want to go on from here "childfree"?

It's spring again. My husband and I are in the midst of adoption proceedings, and we hope to be building a family in the very near future. While the final decision to adopt was made in the last year, the initial steps we took toward adoption went as far back as two years ago. We attended informational meetings; we got on lists; we attended day-long seminars. It seems as if we took out the idea of adoption, held it up to the light, thought about it, and then put it back on the shelf, while we took more tests and kept up the temperature charts. This past year we took it off the shelf and kept it off. I can hardly believe that we're actually preventing conception at this time, too. There'll be no miscarriage this spring.

I miss the hope, the promise, and the dream. But I have a new hope now.

Rosegardens and Fertile Valleys

Sally Chapralis

I "confronted" my infertility by fantasizing. During my treatment, I envisioned myself sitting in the audience at the awards dinner of the All the World Is a Stage Society. Suddenly, my name was announced as the recipient of the Best Supporting Actress in an Unproductive Role. I acknowledged the tribute with a gracious smile. Although disappointed that I had not been reproductive, at least my years of trying had been recognized. A triumph, of sorts.

In my fantasy, I was resplendent in a red-sequined dress with thigh-high slits on both sides, and deep dips in front and back. (You have to show something when you're not "showing.") As I walked through the audience toward the stage, mentally rehearsing my acceptance speech, I serenely bowed to the medical impregnators, anthropologists, and pregnant-career-women-over-fifty contingencies.

Once on stage, I graciously accepted the "That's Life" copper plaque and gushed "Oh, I'm so grateful to so many people for making this impossible. First, Dr. Rosegarden, my psychotherapist, without whose support and constancy I would never have had the courage to pursue fertility. Then, the Fertile Valley Clinic, which orchestrated our participation with sensitivity and the latest in medical technology. Last, but not least, there was my co-star, my husband, Jim, without whose deep love and sperm, this award would have been inconceivable."

It was a wonderful moment, everyone rushing to congratulate me. On my way back to the audience, however, I casually pulled a loose thread on my dress. Suddenly, the sequins trailed behind me on the floor, leaving the glitter and graciousness to the cleaning crew. Which, of course, seemed more like reality.

Reality was bitterness, anger, anguish, incomprehension, a sense of loss so deep and so severe that I was sure that some organ had been removed from my body, leaving in its place a gaping wound, a psychological hurt that no one could ever really see, and a few would even comprehend as little more than self-indulgence.

I am forty and my husband is fifty, and we have been married for twelve years, both for the first time. We wanted children. Within a few years after marriage, after trying most of the contraceptives, we ironically discovered that I suffered from infertility problems. It took me quite a while to digest the ramifications of infertility, but it would take me even longer to realize that I was also neglecting my career, avoiding opportunities because, paradoxically, I might become pregnant. I was only beginning to have inklings of how ingrained my traditionalism really was, despite the fact that I considered myself a liberated woman.

I was in my early thirties when my gynecologist asked me if I were interested in becoming pregnant, and I said yes. And how long had we been trying? Oh, for a few years, but I know these things take time. Yes, but we ought to take some preliminary tests to get on the right track. Oh, I wasn't particularly concerned; after all, I knew about Mother Nature, and she can only be pushed so far by Father Time (chuckle, chuckle).

Several months later, having taken my temperature, noting the peaks and valleys of my menstrual cycle (wondering if the thermometer also reflected my creeping disillusionment and bewilderment); regulating much of our sex life to baby making; and finally, discovering that my husband's sperm were indeed prolific but finding unreceptive quarters, we were referred to a fertility clinic. There, we were asked about our sexual technique, length of our arm spans (it's true), and many other intimacies that would now become part of our record. Surrounded by photos of babies that the clinic had helped to conceive, we were overwhelmed by its cheerleading zealousness but happy that it was there.

I never knew which of the three specialists would see me on any particular day, which further depersonalized a very personal situation. I visited the clinic about four times a month, when "the time" was right, taking drugs to encourage my eggs to give the sperm a fighting chance. Even though I was vaguely aware that I was feeling assaulted by all the explorations into my reproductive tract, I had actually begun to feel as if I were a host personality. There was me, and there was this other world over which I had no control, or, at the very least, had learned to live with.

My husband responded like a trooper to being tapped on the shoulder at 5:00 A.M., before we went to work; being told by me that my temperature said go; and, afterward, driving me to the fertility clinic about forty minutes away, before finally going to his office. (I told my office, when I was late, that I was having dental work.) A fisherman, Jim would encourage me by saying, "Think of my sperm as salmon swimming upstream returning to their spawning grounds." Oh, why not?

Anyway, I thought, after more months of X rays, tests, thermometers, surgical procedures, I don't feel sick. I feel fertile. Then I knew that I had to have a break from this, to try to find myself again. I would return, of course, because our failure could only mean that I wasn't trying hard enough, or I was nervous, or something. I just needed to recharge my batteries, and it would work.

I enrolled in an evening graduate course while I continued to muddle through my career without any defined goals. The course led to a graduate assistantship to work on my M.A. I accepted, became a full-time student, and more officially, a part-time worker. For almost two years, I was stimulated by graduate study, diverted from some real issues, and immersing myself with total abandon in a world that only midterms, finals, and debates about socialism and communism can provide. When I was graduated, I enthusiastically began looking for a new position. But because I still hadn't clarified my goals and needs, I accepted the wrong one for me. Of course, it would only be temporary.

It's not as if I didn't have any ambivalence about having children. Would we be able to juggle childrearing with working, even part-time or with day care? What about our ages? What about everything? I didn't want to be a mother who had decided to become pregnant just to have another experience in life and ended up regarding her "token" as a continual burden. I knew children weren't easy to raise and live with twenty-four hours a day, and the experience could wear on even the most adaptable and resolved parents. But we wanted to create a child, to love it, to nurture it, even to be hurt by its possible "counterdependent adolescent abuse."

I watched the parents I knew as they raised their children, observed the qualities that worked, reflected on those areas in my personality that might be wanting, and ended up feeling better about our ability to handle parenthood. It also occurred to me one day that if I hadn't been so prissy when I was nineteen and the fellow I was dating suggested getting into the back seat of his dad's Ford, that I might be sending some character off to college by now, not contemplating, at the age of thirty-eight, another visit to the fertility clinic.

Which is why, after consultation with my husband, I sought the counsel of Dr. Rosegarden, a psychotherapist. Wading through my fears and fantasies, liberation and tradition, and my midlife crises was no mean feat. But I finally realized that I did want to try to become pregnant one last time. My husband was a little less enthusiastic this time around, understandably, but he agreed to try, too.

For our final attempt, we chose a private specialist not far from our offices. This would, at least, make the experience more convenient, if not more fulfilling. The Fertile Valley Clinic and my personal specialist, Dr. Gardner, did make a difference in my attitude, even though he still posted photos of babies on his bulletin board, and in the waiting room we now appeared even more like grandparents trying to conceive. But my husband was inspired when he was shown a slide of his sperm under the microscope. How long does Dr. Gardner think would be a reasonable time to allow for this last pursuit of our wish? Ten to twelve cycles.

Bolstered by the illusion that medical technology cures everyone, we embarked on the path to fertility one last time. Now, at least, we could artic-

ulate our feelings more clearly and confront the stress of the medical inva-
sions of privacy, the drugs, and our uncertainties. We had each other, we
found continuing sensitivity from Fertile Valley, and I could always talk to
Rosegarden to help allay my qualms. Dr. Rosegarden's office became a
retreat, a way to confront reality and to escape from it at the same time. (I
also had begun to lace my conversations, even in unrelated subjects, with
words such as inconceivable, misconceived, unproductive, counterproduc-
tive . . . you get the picture.)

During this period, I refused to come out of the closet, to tell anyone of
this one last try. If it doesn't happen, I reasoned, what's the point of arousing
interest. Besides, I had become tired and angered by others' insensitive,
intrusive, and "concerned" remarks, and was already wondering if I weren't
abnormally obsessed with this wish. I knew I wouldn't feel less of a woman
without a child, but I did want to fulfill, if I could, a sense of destiny that
only a woman can. Of course, my husband had his fantasies about taking his
son fishing.

By the time my tenth cycle had elapsed, we realized that we simply didn't
have the emotional stamina to continue any longer. We had tried, within
and beyond our expectations. Maybe more trying would have worked and
maybe it wouldn't, but tearfully I thanked Dr. Gardner and said goodbye to
Fertile Valley.

Well, I thought, now you can get on with your life and quit this preoccu-
pation. I was totally unprepared for my unexpected crying spells. Why was
this still happening? Was I truly a neurotic and self-indulgent woman? As I
talked it over with Rosegarden, and then with a remarkable young woman
who had encountered and resolved the same personal experience, and shared
her thoughts and feelings with me and others, I came to realize that I was not
unusual. I had just never faced the real possibility of failure, as flip as I had
been about it. I had spent almost a decade denying this outcome and the
intensity of my wish. Now, I was grieving.

I have no visible injury, no disease, no dear relative or friend to mourn,
only a deep wound in my psyche, a hole where a child might have been. To
many, this seems like a peculiar overreaction. To me and us, and those like
us, it is neither. It is real. I had built a not uncommon fantasy, but a wish has
no form and everything seems to remind you of it. There are no rituals to
guide your mourning, no headstone in the cemetery. As we moved through
all those difficult years—grappling with our goals and unexpected feelings—
the only thing that kept us going was wishful thinking. I, especially, am
learning to bury that dream.

We love each other more deeply today, as a result of this experience and our growth in so many areas. On the other hand, it has taken its toll, and it has forced us to think in new ways about ourselves and our future. We have weathered a significant life crisis and are now using some new found energy to pursue other possibilities. Although I no longer harbor the jealousy and anger (I'm still working on the hurt), I'm hoping time will ease the poignancy I occasionally feel at holidays when we might have been a family—those times when grandparents play with their grandchildren in the park, there's a graduation ceremony, a baby commercial, or even a Saturday matinee when the kids are ruining the movie for you by throwing popcorn at each other.

Everyday, our perspective broadens in new areas, and because conception truly is a miracle, we are gradually accepting our childless lifestyle, redefining ourselves, and moving on.

Not in the Family Way

Maggie Rogers

My mother bore nine children in thirteen years, all by exhilarating natural childbirth. She was nicknamed "Fertile Myrtle," and she never confessed to a moment of discomfort during pregnancy, labor, or delivery. Other women may have had trouble conceiving, or may have lost babies through miscarriage, but in our house, childbearing was one of life's greatest adventures, a heroic odyssey to be embraced—and yes, even enjoyed. Fertility was an unquestioned blessing; motherhood, a woman's inevitable reward.

The childless aunts and cousins who gathered with us at holiday time were certainly odd fixtures in that rollicking household dominated by children. When my own sisters began having children, mostly unplanned, the family tradition of unbridled fertility continued. By now, I am an aunt thirteen times over, preparing to welcome the fourteenth baby. I have spent the last decade watching a parade of little ones burp and crawl and toddle and walk. Last Christmas, I held my three-month-old niece in my arms and sobbed uncontrollably—the sweetness was unbearable, the pain sublime.

Infertility. I am the first woman in my family, or my husband's, to travel this ground, so cold and strange. So it is not usually the family nest, the seven-sister brood, that comforts me on discouraging days; instead, it is the faces and voices of friends who have also had a rocky road to the distant dream of motherhood.

There is the friend and former co-worker who suffered her first miscarriage at my wedding seven years ago. Two more miscarriages and much heartache later, she has adopted two Colombian children. There is the old hometown friend who has spent the last few years being injected, inspected, and dejected (as Arlo Guthrie would say) but who can t seem to get a clear diagnosis. And, of course, there are the brave and wondrous women of my RESOLVE infertility support group who have shared their stories—and listened to mine—for the last year and a half.

We have all surfaced in these last months from the depths of despair with the harrowing memories of nearly drowning—feeling alone, out of control, swallowed in salty, watery whirls. We know what it's like to feel victimized by fate, the medical establishment, insensitive remarks, and our own utter helplessness. No other part of our lives has brought so much chaos and frustration—and yet all the parts of us have been somehow shattered and need repair: our marriages and careers, our passions and interests, our friends and families, our faith, our hope, our self-esteem. That we can laugh about the many indignities of infertility now—that we can swap advice on adoption and even listen to tales of new motherhood—is, to me, a remarkable sign that we are healing. But healing is a slow process, and the scars we bear are not always visible, or quick to fade.

I do have a real scar, a thick pink vertical ridge that slices my belly from navel to pubic bone, a lasting token of my laparotomy last June. I lost a tube in that operation. My surgeon told me that the bands of scar tissue, or adhesions, that she was attempting to remove resembled a "Manhattan traffic jam." I can hardly blame her for sacrificing the tube. Or can I?

One of the peculiar quirks of infertility is that the patient is often as well-informed as the doctor, having researched her condition and explained it to countless internists, gynecologists, specialists, surgeons, and endocrinologists over the years. My general distrust of the medical profession is an "inherited" family characteristic, based in large part on my own woeful early experiences with those people in white. There was a botched tonsillectomy that resulted in messy hemorrhaging. (I can still see the doctor's once-white jacket splattered with my blood.) Far worse, there was the teenage trauma of a burst appendix that was difficult to diagnose. As I lay writhing and moaning, without pain medication, four male doctors carried out a horrible prolonged pelvic exam while a nurse begged them to put me out of my misery. No wonder I have so little tolerance for gynecological exams.

Since then, I have sacrificed my privacy and dignity on the examining table countless times because of infertility. So far, it has all proved, as they say, "fruitless." I suppose if some women lose their faith in God during this process, I have simply reaffirmed my lack of faith in those fallible humans who perform no medical miracles on me. Ah, how I wish believing in miracles could make them happen!

My "problem" can be directly traced to the ruptured appendix and the resulting emergency surgery that left extensive scarring, inside and out. Because the memories of that experience are so painful, I tucked them away in some remote corner of the unconscious, where they gathered dust for years. When I got married in 1980, I wrote to the surgeon whose scalpel and hands had so violated me during adolescence. Did he think that the emergency appendix operation could have in any way affected my child-bearing capabilities? He responded in professional gobbledygook, hemming and hawing that he wasn't sure, but he thought, maybe, that it would not.

Somehow, that doctor's vague assurances were little consolation to me six years later as I lay in the pre-op ward of a Boston hospital, shivering in my skimpy green johnny, awaiting general anesthesia and the operation that would, perhaps, undo the damage caused by the ruptured appendix. As I trembled with anxiety and chill in that room last June, I could not have known that I would emerge from surgery with one Fallopian tube gone and no better than a 20 percent chance of ever becoming pregnant. I only knew that major surgery—that most dreaded of experiences for the person who likes to be in control of her life—was my only chance at all.

In the weeks of recuperation that followed my hospital stay, I relaxed in the comfort of my home, basking in the gifts, care, and attention of my husband, family, and friends. I also grappled with the odds—that the medical miracle I had secretly hoped for might never happen, that the magical presto! pregnancies of my mother and sisters might not be my path to motherhood. And yet, as I wrestled with those demons, I had the dim realization that another miracle had taken place. I was surrounded by people who had stood by me despite their confusion and embarrassment at my "odd" predicament. They had come through my infertility with me, had listened and learned and been transformed by it.

I will not easily forget the day my father carried a supper tray to my bed and stood, bewildered, as I burst into tears at the sight of that meal so lovingly prepared. And how reassuring it is to see two mothers (my own and my husband's) leap across the gap in experience and understanding to lend their support, their strength, and their shoulders when I needed them. (I'd like to be able to muster half their loyalty and wisdom for my own children some day.) I am also finding new ways to approach those sisters and sisters-in-law who move into pregnancy and parenthood so effortlessly (or so it seems). Yes, I still ache over each new baby, but each new mom who acknowledges my pain helps to diminish it.

I must be making progress on this strange road. At New Year's, when I cradled my three-week-old nephew, I didn't feel my heart pound or my eyes water. Instead, I breathed deeply, indulged myself in the soft, sweet pleasure of his touch and smell, and wished for him a world full of promise.

Someday, the promise of motherhood will be fulfilled for me. I suppose we all have to hang onto that golden thread to get us through the tough times. Yes, I grow weary of the dashed hopes every month, but I grow with them, and so does my husband. There is a raw and intense intimacy that we share in those moments of disappointment that is showing me a new side to this commitment called marriage. Our most recent "communion" came during a tropical vacation last winter, when my always-reliable twenty-nine-day cycle lasted an agonizing thirty-six days. He openly wept with me as my period brought us crashing back to reality after days adrift in a fuzzy fantasy world of nursery chimes and baby-soft skin, all mixed up with the exotic setting of palm trees, surf, and sunshine.

By now, that episode has taken its place among the many ups and downs that make up my history of infertility. My husband and I are plugged back into the ordinary events of daily life, and we find some measure of challenge and comfort in the familiar—our jobs, our home, our friends and families, our dog. I find myself thinking less about pregnancy and fertility, and instead, seeking inspiration from life's tiny wonders: a spring snowfall, a call from some long-lost friend, the big hearts and tiny hands of neighborhood children. Each time a friend or sister or mother calls, I hear myself telling them things I didn't know I knew: that I'm getting better at playing this waiting game, that I'm ready for the next move—whatever it is, and that maybe I can even win, scars and all. Each day I seem to shed old skin. And, oddly enough, the bright pink scar on my belly begins to stretch as I grow into my new skin.

Mother's Day

Margaret Rampton Munk

I am afraid
To plant this seed.

The sun is warm,
The earth is rich and ready,
But the days go by,
And still no planting.
Why?

The springtime of my life
Is passing, too.
And ten years' planting
In a willing soil
Have borne no living fruit.
So many times I've waited,
Hoped,
Believed,
That God and nature
Would perform
A miracle
Incredible but common.

Nothing grew.
And often times I feel
The mystery of life and growth
Is known to all but me,
Or that reality
Is not as it appears to be.

I have a choice:
To put aside this seed,
Leaving the planting
To the proven growers,
Pretending not to care
For gardening,
And knowing
If I do not try
I cannot fail.

Or plant,
and risk again
The well-known pain
of watching
For the first brave green
And seeing only
Barren ground.

He also spoke
About a seed,
The mustard's tiny grain,
Almost too small to see,
But, oh - the possibilities!
Those who doubt,
Who fear,
Are not inclined to cultivate it.
But it was to them He spoke.

And God remembered Sarah . . .
Rachel . . .
Hannah . . .
Elizabeth . . .

The seed is in my hand,
The trowel in the other;
I am going to the garden
And the Gardener,
Once more.

12

Pregnancy after Infertility

C OUPLES undergoing long-term infertility diagnosis and treatment come to idealize pregnancy. They imagine that a positive pregnancy test will usher in nine months of joy, climaxed by the miracle of childbirth. Most are ill-prepared for how stressful pregnancy after infertility can be.

Couples who conceive after a history of infertility are extremely anxious. Their pregnancy feels so tenuous, so unreal. Since long-term infertility trains women to be tuned into their bodies, they sometimes know they are pregnant almost from the moment of conception. They don't believe it, but they know something is different.

The moments crawl by in early pregnancy. Infertile women are never two or three months pregnant—they are six weeks and two days pregnant or seven weeks and ten hours along. Infertile women check for bleeding several times a day. Some imagine that they will relax when a heart beat is confirmed, or at the end of the first trimester. Others believe they will be relaxed only after the results of an amniocentesis are in. But the truth is that while it gets easier to believe that a pregnancy is real once it is visible, and, certainly, once movement is felt, the anxiety does not end. Infertile couples know all too well that children do not come easily, and they are constantly anticipating disaster.

Some infertile pregnancies do end in loss. A long period of infertility by no means protects people from the tragedies of miscarriage, ectopic pregnancy, and stillbirth. In fact, infertile women have a higher rate of miscarriage, so their anxiety is not unfounded. Some conditions that are thought to cause infertility, namely endometriosis, mycoplasma, and luteal phase defect, cause particular concern since they are also implicated in miscarriage. Similarly, the surgical repair of tubal problems increases the likelihood of an ectopic pregnancy. And stillbirth, though less likely to be linked to infertility, is cruelest of all when it follows infertility.

But most pregnancies do not end in loss. Even after infertility, the majority result in the birth of healthy infants. It is sad that after all the pain of infertility, most couples cannot settle into a pregnancy and enjoy it. Instead, most find themselves expecting tragedy, always prepared for the roller coaster's next downward spin.

In addition to constant worry, infertile expectant parents often report feeling like "strangers in a strange land." Most are transferred from their infertility specialist at the end of the first trimester. Although some enter "high risk practices," most find themselves in the care of regular obstetricians. While their relationship with the specialist may have been intense and perhaps ambivalent, it was also intimate. Someone who knew, all too well, how difficult it was to achieve this pregnancy, is gone. In his or her place, is a busy obstetrician with a waiting room filled with normal pregnant women.

For women pregnant after infertility, it is difficult to be an ordinary obstetrical patient. Physicians and office staff don't seem to realize that the seemingly uneventful, healthy pregnancies of formerly infertile women are marked by a series of perceived near-catastrophes. The absence of fetal movement for an hour, only a small weight gain between visits, or breasts feeling slightly less full, all set off alarm signals in a patient poised for loss.

To make matters worse, obstetricians frequently say things in innocence that may terrify their patients. For example, a physician reading an ultrasound, or feeling the uterus during an exam may suggest that the patient has her dates wrong—that the baby is really due a week earlier or later than she thought. But infertility patients almost never make mistakes about dates. Since they know precisely when they conceived, they conclude that the physician who questions their dates must be telling them that something is wrong with the baby.

Feelings of isolation often continue into childbirth classes. Some couples are fortunate to be in special classes with others who have experienced infertility or pregnancy loss, but most find themselves amidst budding young couples, with dreams galore and pillows in tow. Often they feel out of place and alone. For even when pregnancy is apparent to the rest of the world, the infertile couple may experience a profound sense of disbelief. When the childbirth class takes the tour of the hospital, visiting the nursery and the delivery rooms, some couples actually wonder why they are there.

Couples who have achieved a pregnancy after infertility often feel that they don't fit in anywhere. Not only do they feel isolated from other expectant parents, but they are also alienated from friends still struggling with infertility. Having been there themselves, they know that their friends are envious, discouraged, and possibly angry. It is painful to tell infertile friends about a pregnancy and, once told, it is hard to know how much distance to keep.

So pregnancy after infertility is a strange state of disbelief and anxiety, of fear and loneliness. There are moments of great joy, but by and large, they are met with caution and suspicion. Because the couple has achieved what they sought for so long, family, friends, and often even the couple themselves, fail to acknowledge that theirs is a lonely journey.

For couples who have experienced pregnancy loss, a new pregnancy is a time of uncertainty. After a single miscarriage, however, anxiety is usually moderate. A couple may worry that something will go wrong again, but unless they are dealing with advanced age, they can usually hold onto the belief that this was a random act of nature. And others are quick to remind them that "it happened for the best."

Couples who have experienced two or more miscarriages, particularly if they were consecutive, are often convinced that something is wrong. Even though the doctors will tell them that having two miscarriages doesn't necessarily mean there is a problem, it certainly *feels* like one.

An ectopic pregnancy is even more cause for alarm because it is frequently a medical emergency, and there is also a risk that it will happen again. Consequently, most women who have had an ectopic pregnancy are monitored closely by their physicians and themselves—to try to avoid a potential rupture.

Finally, there is the tragedy of stillbirth. The couple who have known first trimester miscarriages, usually feel they can relax a bit when their next pregnancy makes it past twelve weeks. The woman who had an ectopic pregnancy can relax when an intrauterine pregnancy has been confirmed by ultrasound, but a couple who has known stillbirth cannot end their vigil. They know, all too well, that a baby can be moving and kicking at thirty-eight or forty weeks and be dead upon delivery.

We have found that there are ways in which physicians and other health care professionals can help during pregnancy after infertility, as well as pregnancy loss. They must accept their patients' anxiety and attempt to ease their worries by offering additional office visits or extra reassurance when appropriate. Infertility patients do need to feel that both they and their caretakers are doing all that they can to protect and nurture their pregnancy.

Physicians and nurses must remember that infertility promotes magical thinking and continued vulnerability to loss. Patients pregnant after infertility are always waiting for something to go wrong. They feel guilty complaining when they don't feel well and they are alarmed if they feel "too well." Anxiety may not be spoken of directly, but may be expressed through excessive phone calls, unusual concerns about nutrition, obsessive questioning, and possibly, requests for additional tests. Caregivers who are flexible and who regard their patients' concerns as legitimate, help their patients to modulate anxiety.

With patients who have experienced pregnancy loss, caregivers should pay particular attention to the point at which the loss occurred in the previous pregnancy. Certainly anyone who has had a prior ectopic pregnancy will be closely monitored early in her pregnancy. But women who have experienced early miscarriages may need some additional attention as well. An ultrasound at eight weeks helps both physician and patient to have a better sense of what to expect.

The physician working with a patient who has lost a baby late in pregnancy, or during delivery, should be prepared for the intense anxiety that she is likely to feel as the critical point approaches. More frequent visits during this time, even if they are not "medically indicated," can help the patient feel some sense of control. It may simply help for her to hear the heartbeat more often. Fears will remain, but they can be somewhat allayed.

The doctor-patient relationship in obstetrics changes dramatically at the moment of birth. Following a normal delivery, it is the pediatrician who is the physician most involved. The obstetrician sees his patient six weeks later and then primarily for routine exams and pap smears. For the infertility patient, this abrupt and dramatic change is sometimes difficult. She has not only lost her relationship with her infertility specialist, but she is also no longer in the special role of the obstetrical patient. Now she really feels alone in a waiting room full of big bellies, even with a baby in tow.

In the pages that follow we include three essays that capture the disbelief and wonder of those pregnant after infertility. Ellen Jean Tepper's first pregnancy ends in miscarriage. Despite her disappointment, she finds her ability to conceive affirming after years of infertility. Rachel Lewis and Risa De Long have successful pregnancies, but each speaks to the fact that people continue to feel infertile, long into a successful pregnancy.

My First Pregnancy

Ellen Jean Tepper

My first pregnancy ended in a first trimester miscarriage. The "products" of a six-year effort at conception landed in Dr. P's trash can along with the mail order catalogues that Dave brought along to distract me. In many ways it was a very sad experience. Still, I look back upon those weeks of early pregnancy as a time of great excitement—and of affirmation. I remember the first week with particular pleasure.

I first suspected that I was pregnant on a beach at Cape Cod. I was there for the day with friends, but after years of infertility, I was more focused on my soon-to-arrive period than on our outing. It was twelve days after ovulation, and since a short luteal phase always causes me to menstruate two or three days early, that July Tuesday was right about time.

Traditionally, I spent days twenty-five and twenty-six in the bathroom, checking for blood. For me it was easier that way. The thermometer told the news too harshly, with no room for error. But a little blood could mean many things—an implantation bleed, some spotting, perhaps. I always gave myself a few hours to accept that it meant what it meant: failed conception.

But I was in a predicament that sunny July day; there were no toilets on the beach. Fortunately, infertility had taught me to approach situations creatively, and this one was no exception. Cautiously, I slipped my finger through the crotch of my bathing suit. Quickly, as though I were scratching. Then I took a discreet look. Clean. Safe on first.

The finger-up-the-vagina-quick-check-test served me well over the next several hours. Again and again, in quick, out clean. Day twenty-six was nearing an end and I was beginning to wonder.

On Wednesday morning I went out running. I have a group of friends that I meet at six A.M. For an hour each day we share the most intimate details of our lives, as well as exchange recipes and movie reviews. But that Wednesday, day twenty-seven, I led two lives. There was regular old infertile me, running along and talking about my day at the Cape, and there was quick-checking, almost-convinced-I-was-pregnant me, now one day early—or one day late.

By Wednesday afternoon, I could stand it no longer. I drove to a pharmacy in a neighboring town, willing to go out of my way so that no one would see me buying a home pregnancy test. Still, I felt exposed. What would the cashier think? The pharmacist? Would they take a look at me and say to themselves, "not her?" Or might they mistake me for someone who had happened, quite by accident, into pregnancy?

As it turned out, I never got as far as the cashier. I examined each test kit, and found that none would work until I was at least nine days late. Since I could barely wait nine hours, I had to find a better way. But what? I couldn't ask for a blood test when I was still officially one day early. And I couldn't ask Dr. P what to do because he'd declared me hopelessly infertile.

By Thursday, day twenty-eight, now on time or two days late, I knew that something was different. I told Wendy while we were running that I suspected I might be pregnant, and swore her to secrecy. Later I phoned Rena and promised myself to stop there. But then there was Sylvia; we'd been through her first pregnancy together and she'd been there when we'd adopted Emily. She was pregnant again and now I was imagining that we might have the chance to do it together. By day's end, six friends knew that I was waiting and hoping.

On Friday I began to think more about those who didn't know what was going on, namely my husband, Dave, and my doctor, than about those who did. I had very mixed feelings about telling each of them. With Dave, I felt it was too much joy to bear. If it were really true, I wanted to save it for his birthday, now eight days away. Also, as long as I held off, I could fantasize over and over again about how I would tell him. There were countless scenarios, each more splendid than the one before. I knew that once I told him, I would have to surrender possibilities.

With Dr. P it was different. It wasn't that I wanted to save the news, but rather I wanted to be sure that I was really pregnant before I called him and embarrassed myself. He had been so certain that I was hopelessly infertile when he told us to adopt. Now I wondered how he would react if I professed pregnancy.

"Hello, Dr. P, I know that you are going to think I'm psychotic, but I think I might be pregnant."

"What makes you think that?"

"Well, I'm fifteen days past ovulation and I've never made it for more than twelve."

"Congratulations. You've treated yourself. But have a blood test on Monday just to be sure."

Somehow I made it through the long slow weekend. "Finger-quick-checks" took up most of the time, and the rest was spent deciding who to tell next. Meanwhile, Dave's birthday was still a good six days off and I was about to burst. Monday morning I could stand it no longer.

"Let's tell Mommy the news." Dave and Emily greeted me when I came in from my running. Some major event, like a poop in the toilet, must have just occurred.

"Well, Mommy has something to tell you." And there it was, spilled out with none of the splendor I'd imagined. Dave just sat there and stared at me in disbelief.

I did have a pregnancy test that day and what I had suspected—but dared not believe for nearly a week—became official.

In my seventh week, I had an ultrasound "just to make sure everything was all right." Until that point, things had seemed to be going well. I was still checking for blood, but I was also craving chopped liver, a hopeful sign, I felt, for someone who had been a vegetarian for twenty years. So when that first ultrasound was "inconclusive," I didn't know how to react. I worried, but I was also very busy being pregnant.

But the ultrasound one week later was a different matter. This time it was conclusive and it revealed that there was no fetal development. A "blighted ovum," they called it to be kind, but the hard, cold facts spoke for themselves. There was a little sac in my uterus and it was empty.

Dr. P preferred to "wait and see," rather than to actively terminate the pregnancy. I suppose he hoped that I would begin to bleed on my own, and in retrospect, I think it would have been easier had it happened that way. But the blood did not come and I continued to have some hope—though it grew dimmer and dimmer—that everything was all right after all.

At twelve weeks something had to be done. I was now convinced that I was no longer pregnant, but it looked unlikely that I would miscarry spontaneously. So we made plans to remove it. What I did not realize ahead of time was that the bloodless, physically painless, antiseptic procedure would seem like an abortion.

Dave and I went to Dr. P's office late one September afternoon. While we waited, I paced about and Dave tried to entertain me with his mail order catalogues.

"How about a plastic cole slaw dish? This one's in the shape of a cabbage."

"This is no time to joke about cold slaw dishes." Actually, I thought that he was pretty funny, but I think that I wanted to be sure that the other people in the waiting room knew I wasn't there for just another Pergonal shot or PK test.

Eventually, the waiting room cleared out and Dr. P was ready to end his day—and my pregnancy. He made quick work of it, vacuuming me out in just a few minutes. Dave saw the placenta, but I saw nothing—no tissue, no blood. A day later I was sorry that I hadn't asked to see it.

With the suspense gone, I was surprised to find that I was not devastated by the loss. Certainly sadness and emptiness were there, but those feelings were also accompanied by a feeling of pride and accomplishment. Whatever would happen in the future, I had now been pregnant. Barren for so long, I now knew that something could begin to grow inside me. I had had a pregnancy test and it had been positive. Yes, for a brief magical moment in time, I had enjoyed chopped liver.

I Never Believed It

Rachel Lewis

I seemed to have had a miscarriage about two months before I conceived my first child, almost a year and a half after we began trying to conceive. My period was ten days late, later than it had ever been. What came out of me did not look like the usual contents of menstruation. After describing it to my reproductive endocrinologist (I didn't have the foresight to save it), he concurred that it was probably a very early miscarriage. He called it a spontaneous abortion.

I was crushed. How could this happen to me? My doctor tried to be reassuring. He said that it was really a very positive sign, that at least I knew I could conceive. I tried to be optimistic and see things his way, though it was difficult to suppress my sadness. It seemed as if I had been trying to get pregnant forever. In retrospect, after having worked for ten years with infertile couples, I now know that I was one of the lucky ones. A year and a half is small potatoes in the cosmic realm of infertility.

Two months after that probable miscarriage, I conceived. When my period was twelve days late I had a beta sub (blood) test for pregnancy. I listened in disbelief when my doctor got on the telephone and said, "Congratulations, pregnant lady!" I can remember asking him if it was possible the lab had made a mistake, or switched my blood with someone else's. He assured me there was no mistake (I imagine he had been asked that question many times before) and also mentioned that the beta sub count was high, indicating a strong pregnancy.

I didn't believe him, not because I am untrusting by nature, or because I had any reason not to trust him. I just didn't believe that I was actually pregnant. Unconsciously, I believed that infertility would be my punishment for having had a relatively easy life. It was also the worst punishment I could imagine. One I felt incapable of surviving.

I also remembered the miscarriage two months earlier, and became certain that even if I were pregnant, I would lose it. I checked periodically for blood. My worries, to some extent, were based on reality. For one thing, I had none of the usual pregnancy symptoms that I had read or heard about: no sore breasts, no fatigue, and no nausea. I kept trying to conjure up those symptoms so I could reassure myself that everything was okay, but no matter how much I poked them, my breasts did not feel tender, and I could not fall asleep in the afternoon. The one change in my body was that I did begin to urinate constantly. I had not known that was common in early pregnancy, so I convinced myself I had a bladder infection that was somehow affecting my reproductive system, and causing my menses to be suppressed. I thus alternated between anticipating a miscarriage, and convincing myself that my bladder was in trouble.

So I drove myself crazy all during my first trimester. When the doctor examined me in my eighth week of pregnancy, and told me that everything was progressing normally, I still did not believe him. I clung fast to the bladder infection theory and reasoned that my uterus was enlarged because I was not able to menstruate due to the infection.

When I was in my tenth week of pregnancy, the doctor heard the heartbeat, or so he said. To me it sounded like a child's choo-choo train. My husband and I were leaving the following week to go on a two-week vacation. I asked the doctor if perhaps he was just telling me he heard it so we could enjoy our vacation. He looked directly at me, and in a kind way assured me he would never do that. It seemed there was no way to convince me that not only was there a fetus, but also that it was developing normally.

I did have moments during which I began to believe I might really be pregnant. During my tenth week of pregnancy, I actually experienced about an hour of nausea around lunchtime. I was thrilled! The timing was unfortunate, however, as I was meeting some colleagues who were taking me out to lunch. When I began to feel better, I didn't know whether to be happy that I could enjoy my meal, or worried that the fleeting nausea was really a fluke and had nothing to do with any pregnancy. I seemed to be getting fatter; certainly I was gaining weight, but that phenomenon was not unknown to me either.

We had told people about the pregnancy early on, though now it seems strange to have done that when I did not believe it myself. I felt like an imposter when friends and family members asked me about my pregnancy or about our plans for the birth. I went through the motions of a pregnant woman—doctor's visits, looking into childbirth classes, even buying maternity clothes. Yet none of it seemed real.

I felt movement in my nineteenth week. At first it felt like a goldfish fluttering around, so I convinced myself that I was wrong about the bladder infection. I decided that I must really have a parasite growing inside me. By the time I was in the middle of my seventh month, the movements began to feel like body parts poking me, or limbs moving. At that point, even my very strong denial (perhaps it was fear), began to fade. I realized that any woman in my condition who still did not believe she was pregnant belonged in a mental hospital.

I began to enjoy my pregnancy more once I believed it was real. Though I must admit that when my son's head emerged from me during delivery, I burst into tears. The moment was highly emotional, but beyond that I cried because the last ounce of denial I had been harboring, had been removed. I finally had the baby for whom I longed and who I never believed would be mine.

Self-Renewing Membership

Risa De Long

Recently, while jogging in my fifth month of pregnancy, I ran into the surgeon who performed my second laparotomy. Although he did not initially recognize me, he informed me that running during pregnancy would be helpful in labor. As he slowed down to keep pace with me, I introduced myself and told him that I had run throughout my first pregnancy. I wanted to tell him more, but before I could do so, he had congratulated me, and run on.

Later, while showering, I thought back on this encounter. How strange that this man, who had operated on me and who was, at least in part, responsible for my son's conception and now for this second miracle pregnancy, did not know me? But stranger still was my sense that he had taken me for a regular pregnant woman.

I am taken for pregnant a lot these days. A full belly camouflages infertility. The baby kicks, my three-year-old reaches out an inquisitive hand to feel it and for a few minutes, I, too, forget.

In some ways it was easier when I was pregnant for the first time. Then I was simply the recipient of a miracle. Hard earned, the result of several surgeries and long, difficult recoveries, but a miracle nonetheless. And after my son was born I returned to my infertility, to questions and concerns about how he would someday become a brother.

Eleven months later, the quiet questions erupted: an ectopic pregnancy, that cruel hoax on those of us who've had our tubes "repaired." I remember the midnight ride to the emergency room. The pregnant teen in the next bay. Later, the all-too-familiar surgical floor. Lying there, before daybreak, I realized that whatever happened in the future, my infertility would remain with me. A self-renewing membership.

Soon we will begin our childbirth refresher course. For a second time, we will join with fertile couples, pillows in hand and dreams intact. We will pant and puff together, reaching for some control over a process that is beyond us.

I am a pregnant, infertile runner. Puzzled and disbelieving, in awe of miracles, I straddle two worlds.

13

Adoption

I N setting out to become parents, few couples initially consider adoption. Most have strong feelings about having their "own" children and regard adoption as something that happens to someone else. They link the drive to be parents with the wish to reproduce, and few imagine the possibility of parenting a child that was born to another.

Adoption is not an issue for most couples. They conceive and carry babies who at birth have Dad's eyes, Mom's mouth, Dad's pitching arm, and Mom's temperament. They never ask themselves if they could love a child they did not bear, perhaps even a child of another race or from another country. They never have to consider taking all their savings to finance an adoption, nor confront fears that they will raise a child who will one day cry out, "You're not my *real* parents."

Couples experiencing long-term infertility or repeated pregnancy loss ask themselves all of these questions—and more. For a few, the answers are easy. Some are clear, from the start, that adoption is an acceptable and viable option. Others feel equally certain that adoption is not for them. But most infertile couples initially approach adoption as cautious and skeptical explorers. They bring with them doubts, fears, prejudice, and misinformation. But often there is also a tiny glimmer of hope.

Infertile couples begin their exploration of adoption in different ways. Some consider it at a time when there is still substantial hope that they will bear a child together. Because they have fears of not having a biological child, they need to have a second choice, and to become comfortable with it long before they are ready to take action. For them adoption is the light at the end of the tunnel—and they need to know it is there.

Other couples go to the end of the tunnel before they look for a light.

They need to exhaust every option, pursue every path to pregnancy, before they can begin to consider an alternative. For them, thinking about adoption and pursuing it may occur simultaneously.

But whether they think about adoption early, during their infertility work-up, or only after all efforts have failed, there are certain questions that prospective adoptive parents ask themselves and others. These are issues that they puzzle over and struggle with before they are ready to adopt.

The questions that infertile couples face when deciding about adoption fall into three groups:

1. Can we love a child that is not "our own"?
2. Is adoption possible for us, financially and legally as well as emotionally?
3. Will there be psychological-emotional problems raising an adopted child?

Each couple explores these questions in their own way, determined in part by their ages, financial situation, religious and cultural backgrounds, and the attitudes of the community in which they live. Let's consider each question individually:

1. *Can we love a child that is not "our own"?* Before answering this question, couples must confront what it will mean to them not to have a biological child. The loss is usually enormous! Most men and women who want to be parents have certain aspects of their heritage that they are proud of and wish to pass on to their offspring. Whether it is curly black hair or exceptional musical ability, is not important. What is important is the intense desire to live on in one's children. Though, of course, no one can ever insure their immortality, couples who are infertile must confront this fantasy much sooner than those who have biological children.

In struggling with this first question, most couples begin by asking themselves whether they could love someone else's child. Many take note of the feelings they have when they are around the children of friends and neighbors, looking for clues for what it would feel like to have one of them as a son or daughter. Later this exploration extends to the community at large. They observe children in parks and playgrounds, walking to school, and riding bikes. They watch and wonder how one falls in love with a child.

The question of whether a couple can love a child they did not bear brings up the question of why they wanted to become parents in the first place, before they knew about their infertility. Some couples never thought much beyond pregnancy and early childhood. They never pictured themselves as parents of a preschooler or even an adolescent. Other couples remember their desire to *parent*, to guide a little person throughout his or her young life—to love and to be loved back. Reconnecting with these nurturing feelings can be a relief to couples considering adoption. They understand that pregnancy and childbirth, though miraculous, are experiences that last nine months, while parenting lasts a lifetime.

Once a couple has made the initial leap of faith and decided that they need not bear a child in order to love it, more specific questions follow. "I could love *someone else's* child but could I love *anyone's* child?" Some begin to question raising a child of another race or religion. Others focus on concerns about inherited illnesses or congenital abnormalities. Some simply think in terms of good genes and bad genes and wonder how you can know what you are getting. Most are troubled by the fact that adoption seems so random.

But most couples find a way to wade through these issues. Some feel that there are things that they can have control over and they decide to pursue adoptions that will maximize this control. Others decide that risk taking is simply a fact of parenting and they conclude that the child they get will be the child they will love.

2. *Is adoption financially and legally possible and are there babies available for adoption?* Once a couple has confronted the basic question of loving a child born to another, there are logistics to consider. Birth control, abortion, and society's acceptance of single parenthood have all reduced the availability of white infants. Social and political discord in third world nations have made foreign adoptions complicated and time consuming. After the long ordeal of infertility, a couple must face new challenges on the road to adoption.

For those with financial resources, the pace of adoption has not changed dramatically. A number of small agencies, nationwide, are placing white, healthy infants in under a year's time. But the cost of these adoptions is very high. They can run between ten and twenty thousand dollars. And because medical and legal costs are ever on the rise, adoption expenses continue to climb.

Couples with limited financial resources are forced to make choices. For some, a foreign adoption is the answer. Foreign adoptions, though still costly, are generally less expensive than private or small agency adoptions. They usually cost under ten thousand dollars. While there can sometimes be delays due to political conditions in the country, or problems with immigration, the wait involved is usually less than a year and a half. In addition, foreign adoptions add cultural dimensions that many couples find enriching.

And often with foreign adoption families have the opportunity to select the sex of their child.

Couples who want to adopt a white baby but whose finances are more limited, are often frustrated in their attempts to do so. Social service agencies have long waiting lists for white infants, many quoting as long as six to eight years. Hence the couple who cannot afford several thousand dollars, or does not want to wait many years for a child, are faced with some difficult decisions. Possibly they can adopt a sibling group, or a child with some medical problem, or one who is legally "at risk," whose birthmother has not yet surrendered him or her for adoption.

Laws vary from state to state, but it is also possible in many states to do an identified adoption, one in which a couple locates a pregnant woman who agrees to surrender her baby to them. Some states, in private adoptions, require the couple to successfully complete a home study in which case a licensed agency acts as a go-between, offering the necessary counseling and legal services. Other states require only the services of a lawyer to legalize the adoption. While costs mount in some of these adoptions, others turn out to be reasonably affordable.

Couples considering adoption are sometimes frightened away by some of the horror stories that they read in the papers or see on TV about adoptions that have fallen through. A couple may learn of a birthmother who changed her mind four months after placement, or a birthfather who appeared on the scene, never having signed a surrender. Tragedies do happen, but a couple can learn what risks are involved in their adoption and make decisions based on this knowledge.

Just as it takes financial and emotional strength to make one's way through infertility diagnosis and treatment, these resources are also needed for adoption. Contrary to public fears, infertile couples are not "buying" babies, or manipulating poor people to give up their children. But those who are informed, are reasonably financially secure, and who have the wherewithal to make their way through the adoption maze, can become parents.

3. *Will an adopted child have social, intellectual, or psychological problems?* Even when couples can see their way clear to adopting, they remain apprehensive about the experience. They may be convinced that they will love the child, but they are less convinced that he or she will love them. Many have fears that the knowledge of the adoption will do irreparable harm to the child. Some fear that their children will search for their birthparents and reclaim them as their own. Others fear the birthparents themselves, regarding them as adversaries. They worry that birthparents will return one day and declare themselves the real parents.

Certainly adoption is not an easy situation for anyone involved. Children do have feelings about it and so do their adoptive parents and birthparents. At certain developmental stages, primarily adolescence and young adulthood, issues of identity are crucial. Children who are adopted may struggle even more during those periods with questions about who they are and to whom they belong. The nature of adoption, however, is changing. These changes promise to make the adoptive experience more comfortable for adoptees, their adoptive parents, and their birthparents.

In the past, little was known about infertility or pregnancy loss. Feelings about these experiences were ignored or dismissed. Infertile couples commonly moved on to adoption having little understanding of why they had not conceived or carried a child. Since a child had not been born, no one understood their loss nor their grief. Consequently, they had little or no opportunity to resolve their feelings of infertility. Thus lingering sadness and anger remained, and often these feelings were directly or indirectly conveyed to the children, who were probably told something like "you were chosen." Worse yet, couples were often advised that adoption would promote fertility, a belief that suggests their problem was psychological in origin. Physicians and/or social workers often implied (or stated outright) to women that a child might somehow alleviate their emotional stress, and allay their deep seated fears about parenting, all suspected to be the cause of their infertility. Infertile women were considered to be unfeminine and hostile toward men, having never resolved their "Oedipal issues." Thus adoptive families were created that were destined to fail.

Today, most couples who are adopting have fully investigated and attempted to treat their infertility. They have intense sad feelings about their inability to bear a child but, in all probability, they have talked out their feelings and explored their reactions. They have the opportunity to grieve that was denied previous generations. Most couples adopt convinced that although it is their second choice, it is their best means to a family. And they can become parents with positive feelings about the process, with true delight in the children that become their "own."

In the past, negative effects of adoption on the adoptee, were compounded by a sense of taboo. Records were sealed and most adoptees grew up with many questions that went unanswered. Their parents, and the social service system in general, dismissed their need to know about their birthparents, and encouraged them to be grateful for the home that they had been given.

Today these sentiments have changed. Now agencies actively promote positive feelings between birth and adoptive parents, sensitizing each group to the feelings of the other. Often the birthparents have the opportunity to select the family who will adopt their child. Sometimes there is even an actual meeting or telephone conversation. Gone are the fears and fantasies about irresponsible, uncaring birthparents and selfish, misguided adoptive parents. In their place is a mutual respect and empathy that is conveyed to the child.

More and more adopted children are growing up in homes that support their curiosity and recognize the need that some adoptees have to search for their biological parents. Many adoptive parents actually assist their children if they decide to search. It is this acceptance of differences—this acknowledgment that adoption does differ from biological parenting—that enables adoptive parents to feel secure in their role. And, in turn, this sense of security allows them to help their children grapple with the issues of identity and belonging that will inevitably arise, especially in adolescence.

Finally, the nature of adoption has changed because it is more visible. In the past, when couples were "matched" with babies, there was no way of visually identifying an adoptive family. While this permitted adoptive families to maintain privacy, it also caused them and others to minimize differences, while promoting a sense of mystery.

Today, many adoptions are visible. It is now commonplace to see white couples with Asian or South American children or racially mixed children. In fact, some women who are married to foreign men find that people assume that their mixed race offspring are adopted. Foreign adoptions have taken the mystery out of all adoptions in our society and helped to make adoption an assumed and accepted way to form a family.

The hardest work for most adoptive parents is the process of deciding whether to adopt, and if so, who, how, and when. Once the decision is made, however, the actual placement is a joyous occasion for most.

Depending on the type of adoption, a couple may have anywhere from a few months' to a few hours' notice that their child is arriving. In foreign adoptions there is often an assignment and a photo, then weeks or months of waiting. In local adoptions, a couple may know that a birthmother has selected them, but they anxiously await her delivery, as they know she may change her mind. Others, pursuing agency adoptions, may simply get a call telling them that they are parents. Consequently, the pre-adoptive period is a time of great uncertainty.

The pre-adoption wait is difficult for a number of reasons. First, infertile couples have already been pushed to their limit by uncertainty. Many have undergone years of treatment that proved unsuccessful. They have turned to adoption hoping for success and having limited ability to cope with further disappointment.

Pre-adoption uncertainty is also difficult from a practical standpoint. It becomes hard to plan for a leave of absence at work, to know when to schedule a vacation, or to plan a job change. From a practical standpoint, it is also difficult to buy a car seat or a crib when there is the possibility that it may sit empty for several months.

Finally, pre-adoptive parents struggle, once again, with their decision. Old doubts return as they wait and wonder if they are doing the right thing. Would it be best to leave well enough alone? Will they get the right baby? And so forth.

On the other hand, sudden parenthood can be magical. After all the years of struggle, adoptive parents are delighted to suddenly find themselves wheeling a shopping cart full of diapers. And there is something exhilarating about awakening to a baby's cries—even at 3:00 A.M.—after years of awakening to a thermometer.

Adoptive parents, like all parents after infertility, soon discover that their infertility has left behind a powerful legacy. Later we will address general concerns that all infertile parents face. However, there are some specific issues that pertain to adoptive parents. Consideration of these issues, prior to adoption, should reduce negative feelings, and enhance the adoption experience for everyone involved.

Almost everyone who parents after infertility or pregnancy loss feels vulnerable. These feelings may be particularly strong for those who adopt. The homestudy itself probes into the private life of the infertile couple. Unlike couples who parent biological children, they are judged as to whether or not they will be sound parents. This judgment renders them at the mercy of their social worker and enhances feelings of helplessness and vulnerability. In addition, uncertainty about their adopted child's future feelings, and how they will respond to him or her contribute to feelings of inadequacy. Insensitive comments from others increase their sense of vulnerability.

Most adoptive parents feel committed to being open about their child's adoption and they reject the notion of secrecy. But early on, they realize that privacy must be distinguished from secrecy. It is not being secretive to smile when someone in a restaurant says "Your little girl looks just like you" or to register your son for nursery school without announcing "He is adopted." There are instances, however, when the border blurs between privacy and secrecy. When the day camp application asks "Is there anything else we should know about your child?" adoptive parents may wonder if there is.

While they are adopting, many new parents develop affection and empathy toward their child's birthparents. These feelings surely help them to bond with their child. But what about the birthparents in years to come? Much has been said about the pros and cons of searching for them, and about open versus closed records, but little attention has been given to the father who watches his four-year-old son blow out birthday candles and thinks of another man, somewhere, who may be remembering the tiny baby he gave up. And what of the novice tooth fairy, who stands in the dark, clutching a tooth and wishing she could send it to someone for whom it would mean so much, someone to whom she is immeasurably grateful. Feelings toward birthparents come up from time to time, often unexpectedly.

All families have religious, ethnic, and cultural heritages that they pass on to their children. But adoptive parents know that their children have other heritages, as well. Adoptive parents look to what they know of their child's birth heritage and sort out ways in which it resembles and differs from their own. They must then decide what to share with their child. Foreign-born children adopted by white American couples, have unmistakable biological heritages. Their adoptive parents usually make great efforts to teach them about the country and culture from where they came. White American babies adopted by white American parents are less different in appearance. Their parents must decide to what extent, if any, they wish to discuss the ethnic and cultural backgrounds of their adopted child with him or her.

Since adopters and adoptees are in the minority in our society, most friends, neighbors, relatives, colleagues, and acquaintances will not be personally involved with adoption. All adoptive parents find that people will say insensitive things, even with the best of intentions. "She looks just like you, she could be your own" or "Do you know anything about her real parents?" It is difficult not to react defensively, and to reply simply, "Of course she is my own," or "We are her real parents."

Like any minority, adoptive families need companions. Developing friendships with other adoptive families diminishes feelings of isolation, for both parents and children. All children want to be "just like everybody else." Those that grow up with friends who are also adopted come to regard adoption as a normal and natural way to build a family. Fortunately, organizations like The Open Door Society promote adoption networks, thus cutting through feelings of isolation that might develop.

For women, in particular, there is a certain clubbiness about pregnancy. While detailed accounts of labor and delivery virtually vanish by the time their children are six months old, references to pregnancy and childbirth come up periodically. For an adoptive mother who feels as if she has finally joined the world of parents these discussions can be painful. She is a mother, but she is not quite in the club.

Biological mothers and their children begin as one and move toward separateness. Adoptive families begin with separation, move toward oneness, and then toward separateness again. It is difficult for all parents to let go, as separation means loss. But sometimes adoptive parents experience this loss more intensely because they did not begin with an assumption of oneness. The bonds in adoption are strong and born of great commitment, but they differ from those that exist, without question, in biological relationships.

Because they did not pass their genes onto their children, adoptive parents may feel additional need to shape their child's environment. But what they find, along the way, is what all parents discover: children are who they are. Surely children have some inherited traits and talents, and others that are environmentally influenced. But, by and large, children come into this world with personalities and temperaments that are distinctly their own.

In his 1964 book, *Shared Fate*, H. David Kirk looks at patterns of adoptive family relationships. He suggests that parents can either reject differences between themselves and their adopted children or acknowledge them. Rejection of differences, though necessary and helpful at times in some aspects of parenting, proves to be the least adaptive means of coping. By contrast, couples who comfortably acknowledge differences and embrace them, seem to have warmer, more empathic relationships with their children.

The essays and poems in this chapter offer various glimpses of the adoption experience. In her poem, "Mother," Marcia Lynch expresses fears that the bureaucracy involved in her foreign adoption will prevent her from ever becoming a mother. Sharon Jette describes her process of deciding to become an adoptive mother—how she came to see that although it was initially her second choice, her child would always be "first best" in her heart.

The next three pieces in this chapter deal with feelings toward birthparents. In her poem, "The Mother of My Child," Judith Steinbergh "dreams" of her child's birthmother. In "I Spy," Gabriella West recounts the unusual opportunity she had to "spy" on her son's birthparents, and the feelings she had in doing so. Jean Lindquist in "You Are Our Parents," shares with us the perspective of an adult adoptee whose successful search for her birthparents provided the missing link in her own identity development. In

"The Biggest Decision of My Life," Camille Wisniski presents a fascinating drama of a couple who adopted three special needs siblings. Ellen Sarasohn Glazer responds to the question, "Will an adopted child ever feel like our own?" in her essay, "A Child of Our Own: Some Thoughts about Birth and Adoption." And the final piece in this chapter is a poem by Fran Castan. "The Adoption" captures the memory of that magical moment when mother and baby bonded together in love and truly "adopted" each other.

Mother

Marcia Lynch

This may never come to be, I fear:
the child who turns to me, who calls one day,
"Mother, mother," words I long to hear.

Son or daughter, olive-skinned, or fair,
or tan—a healthy child is what I pray.
But this may never come to be. I fear

the long thread of dreams will reappear
where countless orphans mouth in silent play,
"Mother, mother." The words I long to hear,

silent as leaves, lift high with the wind. They veer
beyond my reach. I am such easy prey
to the one who's never come to me. I fear

bureaucracy will make me wait another year,
pregnant in papers that ask what I will pay
to be a mother. Oh, Mother, the words I long to hear

are the same I cried to you. Mother, say
the story has a happy end. I'm afraid
this may never come to be. I fear
"Mother, mother"—the very words I long to hear.

Adoption: Second Choice or Second Best?

Sharon Jette

I recall approaching adoption most tentatively at first, still trapped within the cycles of fertility failure and unwilling to hope for any alternative path to parenthood. When the caseworker for my first homestudy asked if I believed adoption to be a "second choice," I had no idea how to handle her question. Overwhelmed with anxiety, and afraid to give the wrong answer, I dissolved into tears. Her question echoed in my mind for weeks before I faced it squarely: was adoption a second choice or a second best solution for me?

At the time, I was pursuing medical treatment and adoption concurrently. In fact, on one particularly memorable day, I caused a minor traffic accident while racing from a morning medical appointment to an afternoon adoption interview. My heart as well as my hopes were divided between two pathways, so that adoption indeed felt "second best," when that critical question was asked of me. The experience of infertility seemed to have crushed my self-confidence and replaced it with feelings of jealousy, suspicion, and fear of failure. I could no longer be objective about myself or about anyone else. I worried about my ability to be an adoptive parent, and I was afraid to trust my caseworker.

I recall dreaming as I awaited placement of my child. Ideally, I wanted this child to know that the best possible plan had been chosen for her. Silently, I pledged to be the best possible parent. But prior to her arrival, I resented most bitterly the process of having to prove myself a worthy and competent parent in advance. It seemed as if I was asked to prove myself a good driver without ever having sat behind the wheel of a car. Despite my nervousness, I believed I would do a good job. But how could I claim success before the fact?

Feelings of inadequacy accompanying infertility also tested the strength of my marriage; as in most cases, we did not reach a spontaneous or simultaneous decision to adopt. My husband expressed a willingness to consider alternatives well before I neared the completion of our infertility treatment. When my husband spoke of international adoption some two years before I could consider it, it seemed to me that he was abandoning our mutual goal of pregnancy. I felt terribly guilty as I questioned my inadequate abilities to parent a bicultural family. It was the occurrence of a tragic event—the murder of John Lennon in New York City—that inspired me to choose adoption. Listening to replays of his popular song, *Imagine*, I found the courage to be different, and to imagine myself parenting a mixed family without regard to artificial boundaries of race or color.

Once resolved in my own decision to adopt, I was better prepared to handle the few, but inevitable opinions from others that our decision was second best. Family and friends needed time to adjust and to confront their own fears and bigotries. The easiest reply was to laud our humanitarian intent to save a child from hunger and disease. But failure to conceive had left me fearful that I would fail the homestudy, fail to adopt—or worse—fail to nurture this gift of a child. I felt that few others could comprehend these pre-adoptive fears of mine.

The final challenge I faced was to integrate our child's heritage with that of our families, to believe in my heart that she truly belonged to us. In my husband's family two heirlooms were kept for our children. A delicate christening dress was folded in tissue and carefully wrapped to await our first-born. I asked myself again and again if I could place an adopted child in this dress and celebrate her arrival with joy. After some time, I could clearly answer "yes," knowing this child arrived via our second choice route, but that she was "first best" in our hearts. I could also imagine rocking her in my husband's family cradle knowing she would be secure in our home and in our lives.

Although often used interchangeably, the terms "second best" and "second choice" are not identical. *Second choice* acknowledges the fact that infertile couples first pursued pregnancy; adoption is a second choice for those of us who adopt for reasons of infertility. Yet adoption need not be *second best*, a term that denotes a lesser value on both parent and child. Indeed, it becomes the best possible and most realistic pathway to parenthood for so many infertile couples.

Now, after two successful adoptions and with the benefit of hindsight, I understand better the caseworker's need to determine if I could overcome the "second best" feelings of inadequacy that are the byproduct of infertility. As a parent, I now understand that my adopted children will most probably struggle with their identities. It is especially important that they feel secure in my belief in them as my best possible children. And that belief, combined with our deep love for them, shall be the heirlooms—along with the christening dress and the cradle—that they can pass on to their children.

The Mother of My Child
for the birthmothers of my two adopted children

Judith Steinbergh

a baby fills my dream womb
like a full moon opened by tide

it is there
sudden as dawn
spinning toward me

> the mother of my child
> is heaving tonight
> like a spring mountain
> winter is thawing
> from her insides
> she will give up the child
> she will contract
> into a young girl
> wondering at this flood
> wondering at this lost
> territory

a woman calls
official as a head of state
to declare
she is keeping her child
that is all
that is all
the phone withers
in my hand
sleep writhes
out of my skin
like a snake
I am new
to such night cold terror
the breaking of treaties

> the mother of my child
> is a child
> she wimpers
> she can t remember
> why
> she has handed
> the moon out of her sky
> like a cookie

I reach out
she is smiling
she hands me her motherhood
like a birthright
it is my child
golden as a canyon
for a moment guilt
slides away
like a sweet rain

> now the darkness
> covers her with ivy
> over her flat belly
> over her knuckles
> over her eyes
> feeling
> its persistent claw
> she wills the slow wall
> to blot her growing hollow

I Spy

Gabriella West

My son, Jesse, was born to another couple and came to us when he was four days old. He came so young and so quickly—it took us five months from the time we decided to adopt until placement—because we did what is known as an "identified adoption."

Identified adoption involves locating a pregnant woman who plans to surrender her infant and hoping she will agree that you should be the parents of her baby. It is not an easy process. First, the couple must compose a letter to be mailed to hundreds of friends, associates, physicians, and lawyers. The letter should have broad appeal since you don't know who will be reading it or what will matter to them. It's easy to know what to leave out, but not so clear what to include.

Then there is the telephone. Since the letter uses only first names and includes no specific identifying data, the phone should be a separate unlisted line. People who know pregnant women, or the women themselves, can call the couple directly or can contact their agency. In either event, anonymity is preserved on both ends.

But this is not intended as a story about how we adopted and so I won't make a short story long. Suffice it to say that Paul and I managed to compose a letter, take a nice photo, and survive days upon days when the phone did not ring. When it did ring it was Jesse's birthmother. She was eight months pregnant and determined to surrender. She and her boyfriend, the father, had seen our letter and had decided that we would be the parents.

It all sounded too good to be true. Tense weeks followed, awaiting her labor and delivery, but all went remarkably well. The birthmother phoned us when Jesse was born and told us that we had a son. The agency cooperated and moved things along so that he could be placed directly from the hospital. The greatest gift that I had ever received came from a stranger whom I had never seen, whose name I did not know.

Now much is made these days of the adoptee's need to search—not to find other parents but to "close the circle." But no one talks of the adoptive parents' feelings toward the birthmother: gratitude, curiosity, a need to simply know a name or a face. During Jesse's early weeks I thought often of his birthparents. I hoped that they were happy. I wished that they could see Jesse smile.

When Jesse was six months old the unexpected happened once again. Through a series of coincidences too complicated and too confidential to explain, I learned that Jesse's birthparents would be visiting my next door neighbors. I know that that sounds hard to believe, and it was, but so was his arrival.

There I was with the opportunity to see my son's birthparents. But should I take it? Part of me said that I was invading their privacy. It felt unfair to them. Disrespectful. But another voice said "Go for it. You're in the right place at the right time. You're about to have an experience that will be of great help to you—and to Jesse."

I was nervous, but convinced. I stood back from the window, just far enough so that no one could see me. I felt as if I were in an episode of "I Spy." As the car door opened, Jesse stirred from his sound sleep. My heart pounded. I thought that he knew they were near. Then he rolled over and continued his sound sleep. I continued my watch.

Jesse's birthfather was the first one out of the car. And there he was—the big person that my little person so closely resembled. My knees felt weak. I couldn't quite believe how much they looked alike. Jesse will be tall and handsome.

But it was harder watching her. There was the woman who had carried my son. She was the one who had truly given him life. She didn't look much like Jesse but she was very pretty. Not to sound immodest, she looked like me.

He and she, whose names I do not know, were laughing and talking. I could see that they were happy. I am sure that they carry some pain for having surrendered Jesse, but that day, through my window, I saw happiness. This was a great relief to me.

When Jesse awoke I held him tight. Tighter than ever before. I now had a picture in my mind's eye that I could share with him. It would make things easier for both of us.

I expect that someday Jesse will want to close the circle himself. I anticipate that he will want to search for his birthparents. If he wants, I will help him in the search. My "I Spy" memory will help along the way.

You Are Our Parents

Jean Lindquist

I am an adult who was adopted at eleven weeks of age. In the 1950s, agencies tried hard to match families ethnically and physically, consequently my Norwegian/Northern Italian biological background suited my Dutch/Swedish adoptive parents. Acquaintances have always remarked on how much like my parents I look. I mention this because I wonder if my childhood experiences would be significantly different if I had looked quite different from my family. Also in the 50s, agencies were very secretive about providing adoptive parents with information. In my case, there was some verbal exchange of ethnic background information, a little bit about the birthmother being young, but very little else.

As a young person, I don't recall experiencing negative stereotyping or slurs on my personhood for being adopted. For much of my childhood being adopted seemed, on a conscious level, to be a minor fact of my life. As I reached my teens I began to think and wonder more about this missing nine prenatal months and the lost eleven weeks of my life spent in foster care. During my twenties I re-examined my childhood from the perspective of an adopted person. I began to realize that some of my behaviors and feelings were different from my friends', that I carried particular fears that were bigger and darker than theirs appeared to be, and that certain things about their identity that they took for granted were major unknowns for me. Their lives, unlike mine, were a continuous thread from the moment of conception to the present. I began to think more and more about being adopted.

I was taking a course in college called "Transracial Adoption," which stirred up many feelings and questions that I had never known were inside of me. I went home and asked my mother a number of questions such as: Do you or anyone else know anything more about my story? My mother told me what she remembered, but it was all very sketchy. Soon after this she wrote to the social worker who had placed me and requested more information. The worker responded saying she would be glad to share what non-identifying information she could, but wanted to speak with me in person. As she was on the opposite coast this option was not available to me for several years.

When I had the opportunity four years later to meet the social worker, the first thing she said to me was, "You look just like your birthmother." It was an astounding moment. In a way it was the first time that I had any concrete proof that I existed prior to my adoption. She answered my lists of questions as best she could and provided me with much information during our visit. It was lucky for me that she was still working for the same agency and was so willing to help me. In many ways I wanted to find my birthparents even more, but I also had received so much information that I knew it would take a long time to assimilate it into my image of myself. For some time I just kept marveling that *someone* knew me before; that it was true that I existed.

As I entered my thirties I decided I was ready to actively search for these birthparents, and I became involved with the growing adoptee's roots and rights movement. During this time I continued to develop opinions about how the experience of loss, disruption, and adoption colored my life experience.

It is unfortunate that our language has only these words—mother, father, parents—to describe two linked but separate relationships. There is the relationship of giving birth to a person who carries on a biological connection, and there is the relationship that grows and develops over the months and years of childrearing. Both relationships legitimately deserve to be termed parent-child, though most people are biologically connected to the children they raise. But for those of us who are adopted, these separate relationships exist within separate people.

In my experience the fact of being adopted is not the problem. What problems I have experienced, and can trace back to my early childhood, are not because I was adopted. Adoption gave me a home; the active love and support of parents who think the world of me; a brother, aunts and uncles, and cousins; a connection to the present and a base for my future. Rather, the difficulties I faced as an adult stemmed from the legally enforced secrecy mandated by society, which shrouded and obscured my awareness of my early existence. This secrecy forced me to bury inside the early losses I felt, and although I did not know it at the time, it prevented me from resolving them.

Looking back at my childhood and young adulthood, I would describe the overriding difficulty as being one of confusion. I didn't know where, or if, I belonged. Where did I come from? Who did I belong to? Could "They" take me away? Could I really stay with my family forever? Was I born? Who would I be if I had stayed with my birthmother? Was I who we said I was? Why did my birth certificate lie? Who was I before I was adopted? Did I have some fatal flaw that caused me to be sent away? Were some parents more real than others? Was there someone I really looked like? Did anyone remember me when I wasn't around?

I have always been careful not to inflict myself on others, not to intrude where I might not be welcome. I have spent an inordinate amount of energy trying hard to be very good. I have always had a difficult time leaving my parents or parting with friends. I was mainly afraid that I would never see them again. I am now confident that these concerns, usually unacknowledged, were connected to the loss and disruption I experienced as a baby.

As an adult, it has been a challenge to see myself as the competent, intelligent, respected, and loved woman I am. It's as if the reality of who I am was driven into the drifting sand of secrecy and unspoken loss. The sands would shift at unpredictable times, mystifying my friends and associates and confusing me with self-doubt.

At thirty-one I was ready to face the self-doubt and vanquish it at whatever cost. I began an active search for my birthparents, with the assistance and support of my mother and a network of friends. Part of the motivation was that my father had died, and I realized that I would be upset with myself if I waited too long and found that my birthparents were not alive. The details of the two-year search and consequent reunion are the stuff of which movies are made. I struggled not only with the objective difficulties involved in searching, but also internally: hope, eagerness, disappointment, ambivalence, fear, worry, doubt. But I persevered and one of the unexpected prizes from this quest became the awareness and growth that my family and I experienced together.

Much of my struggle during the two years of persistent, active searching was that I couldn't keep the questions quiet, I couldn't *forget* I was an adopted person. Every step I took forced me time and again to face the possibility that this step would provide the key to actually locating my birthmother. Therefore, before I could take that step I had to prepare myself for finding her. Would she remember me? Acknowledge me? Ignore my letter? Welcome me? As each step was not the final one, but merely one step closer, I had to still my combined excitement and fear and overcome my disappointment. In a way it was re-experiencing the original loss over and over.

When I finally found her, I couldn't believe it. It seemed so sudden! Even though I'd been looking forever, a part of me never expected to find her—certainly not *today!* In our first phone call she was warm and welcoming. The only thing I can remember of the conversation were her opening words, "You must have so many questions and I want to answer them all." My only question was, "Is it really you?" "Yes."

We met the next weekend. I was trembling and lightheaded as I went to our agreed upon reunion. All I had ever wanted was the chance to see her once. I had no expectations or requirements of her except that one—it was my right to meet her. I had no expectations about the future. I knew I had no way of knowing, before meeting her, what sort of relationship, if any, I would want or would be appropriate. I could only ford one river at a time. I was about to meet the irrefutable proof that I was born, that I had existed before eleven weeks. Would I see myself? Would I see myself in twenty-one years? I was about to find a person I had been seeking, consciously and unconsciously, for most of my life. Would I be late and miss the rendezvous, foiled once again?

No. We met under the big clock at Grand Central Station in New York City. We embraced, stared, walked, and talked for eight hours. I met my half-sister. She met my mother. We talked and talked. We compared hands and feet, legs and waists. We looked and looked. By the end of the weekend we were all exhausted!

Three months later I met my birthfather. What excitement to see him get off the airplane! He recognized me immediately—I looked so much like his lover of thirty-four years earlier. I saw a warm, open, affectionate, sentimental man who looked familiar. We walked and talked and held hands for six hours. Again, by the end of the weekend we were exhausted!

But I had heard two sides of a story. A story that was a part of my story. I had seen myself reflected in the looks, gestures, complexion, and body type of two unrelated people. I looked like a combination of them.

And as the months passed the shifting sand found its bedrock. I came from somewhere. I was wanted—not only by the family that had raised me, but also by those who had relinquished me. It was not that they wanted me back—that decision was in the past—but that I was wanted. I had done nothing to cause my relinquishment. I was free of the questing child trapped inside of me. And because these questions were finally resolved, I could finally belong fully to my adoptive family.

That Mother's Day, my mother and I spent a special time together, honoring the years we had shared. She told me that for the first time ever she felt like a real mother. She confessed that all these years she had felt like an imposter. My heart broke for the cruelty of a world that convinced this dear mother that she wasn't a "real mother" because she didn't give birth to her children. I cried with joy that my search freed both of us from the grip of self-doubt and silence.

I now speak with the voice of one whose unspoken questions of a lifetime have been answered, who has experienced the need to belong, who has witnessed the void of a birthparent and the doubt of a parent.

You have a right to have us, your adopted children. We need to know we belong with you. You are our real parents. And the knowledge that we belong together can only make it safer for us to embark on the search for where we came from. It is our right to know both these things and it is that knowledge—that we came from somewhere and that we belong together—that will make us family.

The Biggest Decision of my Life

Camille Wisniski

"Yes, Louise, I can talk now," I looked out from my teller's window. Five people were in my line and others were advancing rapidly in the noonday rush. But I had waited too long for this phone call and I wasn't waiting any longer.

Louise, our social worker from the adoption agency, said, "Are you sitting down?" Now I was really excited.

"Do you have a child for us?" I asked.

"Not one" she said, "I have three."

At that point I believe I was speechless, so she just continued: "Ages two, four, and six. The two oldest are girls, but there are three problems to consider. First, there are three kids and you were only planning on one. Second, there's a legal risk: the parents' rights have not been terminated as yet so the children are not legally adoptable. And third, there's a medical problem. The two youngest ones have a mild case of a bone disease called Osteogenesis Imperfecta (brittle bones). It's an inherited disease and although the oldest doesn't have it she could pass the disease on to her children." She finished by saying, "I know this is a big decision and I don't expect an answer today. I'll give you the weekend to think it over and you can call me on Monday to let me know what you decide."

After I hung up everybody came over to find out what was going on.

They were all very excited for me. They knew how long we had been waiting to adopt a child. They suggested I call Bob and let him know the good news.

I had forgotten all about Bob. I was still in a state of shock and I really didn't know what to do next. When I finally calmed down enough to dial the phone, I gave Bob a call. He was annoyingly calm and practical as he said, "We'll talk about it when we get home, but don't get too excited until we find out all the details." That was so typical of Bob; he always managed to bring me back down to earth and get me thinking sensibly again. He is not the one to jump the gun; I usually am. He's very analytical and has to know all the facts before he'll even show he might be interested. That's why I was surprised by his encouragement and enthusiasm in the days that followed.

When Bob got home that night I was all excited again. We discussed the pros and cons of these three children all night long. The fact that there were three was not really a problem. We had always wanted a big family, but we thought that was impossible at this stage of the game. Besides, when you're going to adopt, whether you adopt one or three, what's the difference? (Boy, did I have a lot to learn. There's a big difference.)

My big concern was the bone disease. We had definitely let the agency know we were not capable of taking on handicapped children. I always marveled at those people that could do that, but I was definitely not one of those people. Just what kind of problems did we face? Then I made the mistake of looking the disease up in the encyclopedia. It described this disease in detail, stating that, in severe cases, children born with the disease can have every bone in their body broken during the birth process. Many die at birth as a result of these breaks. But of course, these children have a very mild case. Emphasis on the word *mild*, I said to myself.

Bob's biggest concern was the legal risk. He was afraid we would grow to love them and then the state would take them away. That was definitely something to consider.

This had to be the longest weekend of my life. With Bob's encouragement, I started calling people. First I called my sisters. They were just thrilled, and the more I talked about it, the more excited I got. I had to work myself up to calling my parents. I imagined they would think we were crazy even to consider three kids, but my mother was very good. She simply said, "The decision is yours, but whatever you decide, we will support you."

I was a little disappointed in her lack of enthusiasm, but the next day my mother called back to say she couldn't sleep all night she was so excited. She felt this was meant to be and asked what they could do to help. That was it, my sign from God. I always felt my mother had a "hot line" to God and she would be the one to tell me when the moment was right, and now she did.

Monday finally arrived. I called Louise bright and early and I'm sure she could sense my excitement over the phone. She let me know right away that we were only one of five couples being considered for these children, so the decision wasn't entirely ours. We set up an appointment to meet with the children's case worker, Barbara. On Wednesday, she and Louise would come out to the house and discuss all the details. I couldn't believe how quickly things were moving.

There was a lot to be done if we were to get these kids. We didn't even have a bedroom for one child, never mind three. We had built our own home, with the help of family and friends. It's our dream house (we dream it'll be finished some day); unfortunately, it wasn't complete at this time. We didn't have any of the bedrooms upstairs done. Our bedroom was set up in the library on the first floor. We didn't have any heat upstairs, we didn't have any closets done, we didn't even have any toilets up there. So we certainly had our work cut out for us. I was just hoping the caseworker had a good imagination and could imagine these rooms complete.

We went to the bank right away and took out a loan to buy all the lumber we needed to finish the upstairs. We also bought stain and varnish and ordered the heating supplies, toilets, and also all the carpets. (How's that for positive thinking?) We were ready.

Barbara and Louise arrived on Wednesday. Barbara had brought tons of pictures with her. No doubt about it, the kids were adorable. The oldest was Heidi, then there was Caroline, and the little boy's name was Bobby. (Another sign from God?) Bobby even looked like Bob. It was incredible.

I sat there taking in all the information Barbara had. Heidi was five when she was placed in the foster home. She was presently in kindergarten for the second year because they didn't feel she was ready for first grade. Her birthday was St. Patrick's Day and she would be seven then. She didn't have any serious behavior problems, but she did have an articulation problem that she would probably overcome with proper speech therapy.

Caroline was three when she was placed in the foster home. She was now four and very bubbly and active. She loved to talk. She had had two broken bones in her life. A broken arm and a broken leg.

Bobby was eight months old when he was placed. The state had been following his progress and decided to remove him from his mother's care when they saw signs of "failure to thrive." That meant he was physically and mentally underdeveloped. When they placed him in the foster home where he received proper food and attention, they found he began to grow and progress normally. He'd had one broken leg in his life. Of course, he'd only been walking for about a year.

By the time Barbara left, Bob was certain these kids were right for us, and I was uncertain of everything. I just wasn't sure I could handle all that responsibility and if I couldn't, what would the results be?

When Barbara left she said she still had four more couples to interview, but she felt very good about us and she would let us know in a week what her decision was. I felt as if we were in a beauty contest. The only difference was, there was no first runner up; either you won or you lost.

In the week that followed, we must have called Barbara every day. We wanted her to know we were interested. (That was Bob's idea.) During this time, I have to admit I was pretty certain Barbara would choose us. I was so excited, I could hardly get through my work day.

Then the day finally arrived. She said there would be a meeting at 9:00 A.M. and she would let me know either way by noontime. I couldn't even do my work. Every time the phone rang, I jumped. Then noon came, then 1:00, then 2:00, then 3:00, then 4:00; then it was time to go home. By the time I left, I was in tears. I knew she hadn't called because it was bad news. When I got home I was really depressed. I decided to work upstairs. I mean, even if we didn't get these kids, we were bound to get a child sooner or later and we would need a room to put it in.

Then the phone rang. It was Barbara. "Sorry I didn't call sooner, but I got tied up." She said, "If you still want the kids, they're yours."

"Of course we want them," I shouted into the phone. I couldn't believe it. I never had such a swing of emotions in my life. I went from totally depressed to totally delirious in a matter of seconds.

I was anxious to hear what the next step was, so Barbara explained. First, she would arrange for us to meet the kids at the foster home. Then she would bring the kids out to our house for a visit. After that, she would bring them out and leave us alone for a few hours to see how we did. And, finally, she would bring them for a weekend and then, on Monday, we would return them to the foster home so the kids could say their *good-byes*. Then they would be ours for keeps. My head was in a spin. That meant that in a matter of weeks I would be the mother of three. Wow!

For the next couple of days I was so excited I could think of nothing else but the kids. We had set a date to meet them on the following Wednesday. I was really flying high when Bob came home one night. He said his sister had called him at work. She had been to see her doctor (an orthopedic specialist) and while she was there she mentioned our situation. The doctor said he had seen patients with this disease before and that they can become deformed from all the breaks. They're usually very small in stature and there's a possibility they could become blind and deaf. They can also develop another bone disease when they get older where the weight of their bodies causes the bones to crush. And, he added, if his children were considering adopting these kids, he would definitely tell them not to.

Bob said, calmly, "I told my sister we knew all those facts, but we feel we can handle it."

At this point, I was hysterical. I knew I couldn't handle all that despite what Bob said. I didn t sleep all night. I couldn't get this picture out of my head of children who were blind and deaf in wheelchairs. Not at all what I had in mind for my family. I had to wait until the next day before I could call Dr. Roe (a specialist in this disease). My voice was still shaking when I called.

He was very patient and understanding. He explained very carefully that one of the characteristics of this disease is that the whites of the eyes are a light blue, but this does not affect the childrens' vision.

He also explained that when such children reach adolescence, there is a chance that a tiny bone in their ear might break causing some hearing loss, but definitely not deafness. And as far as the bones' being crushed, this is a common condition that occurs in many people in their late forties or early fifties. It isn't nearly as devastating as it sounds and it may not even occur in such mild cases as these children had. He finished up by saying that this disease does improve with age and that, once the children reached adolescence, the worst would be over.

Needless to say, I was very relieved. I called Bob right away to tell him the news. We were both very excited and ready to get on with the next step, which was to meet the children.

Well, Wednesday finally arrived and we were ready to meet the kids for the first time. I had made some Valentine cookies for them and I was so excited I could hardly stand it. It was an hour-and-a-half drive to the agency, but of course we got lost, so it took us an extra hour. By the time we got there, I was a nervous wreck. Barbara took us from the agency to the foster home, about a fifteen-minute ride.

When we arrived, we could see these little eyes peeking out from the front window. I guess they were as anxious as we were. I had really expected this to be a magic moment for all of us. Just like in the movies, our eyes would meet and we would immediately fall in love and hearts would appear in the air and music would play. That's not the way it happened at all.

My first thought when I saw the girls was, "They don't look anything like their pictures." Their hair was all knotted and tangled. Heidi still had a barrette in her hair from the day before and Caroline's hair was falling in her eyes. They had dressed themselves that day, and that was fairly obvious just by looking at them. The girls were so excited that they could not control themselves. They were everywhere. But, that was not the worst of it. When Heidi began to talk, I realized I could not understand much of what she was saying. The "articulation" problem seemed more severe than I expected.

Barbara introduced us as Bob and Camille, but the kids knew Barbara was looking for a new mommy and daddy for them, and by the time we left they were calling us "Mommy" and "Daddy" without any encouragement from us.

Bobby had been napping when we arrived, but the foster mother brought him down for a little while so we could see him. She plopped him down in front of the TV and he didn't move. Bob finally reached over and picked him up and put him on his lap and tickled him. Bobby really seemed to enjoy it. The foster mother was surprised, she said Bobby never liked to go to anyone he didn't know well. I have to admit this was the highlight of the whole day: just watching Bob with Bobby.

When we got ready to leave, the girls hugged and kissed us and told us they loved us. They asked us if we were going to be their new mommy and daddy. We said, "Well, maybe," but neither one of us felt comfortable saying *yes* or *no* without discussing it with the other one.

It was a long and tearful ride back home. It seemed that we were facing a lot more problems than I had expected, and maybe I had counted too much on that "magic moment," so I was naturally disappointed. I felt confused and uncertain. By the time we got home, I was a wreck. I didn't want to talk to anyone. I went right to my room and I cried and I prayed. I told God I needed a sign and He had better be specific. I would have settled for a burning bush or a dove or anything that would let me know that this was the right choice to make. Nothing, not even a clash of thunder.

Then Bob came in the room. I could tell his heart was aching. He knew the decision was mine and so did I. But when I saw his face, I realized there was only one choice. I looked at him and I said, "I've decided. We're going to take the kids." And suddenly, I felt a great relief, like a great weight had been lifted off my shoulders and I realized that was my sign. It wasn't a burning bush or a clash of thunder or anything dramatic like that. It was simply a feeling, very subtle, but very specific.

Well, it's been a little over a year since the kids have come, and in the past year we've had four broken bones (one during a blizzard), three cases of chicken pox, two cases of bronchitis, one unexplained rash, one fantastic Christmas, three beautiful birthday parties, and our best vacation ever in Florida. We've had a visit from the tooth fairy. We've carved pumpkins and gone trick-or-treating. We've had emotional turmoil and total chaos. But we've lived through it all, thanks to the support of a wonderful family and some truly fantastic friends. We've also had two caseworkers who have always been there when things got out of control. I've met some incredible people through the school and counseling who have shown care and understanding. But most important of all was the support of a wonderful husband. He's helped me to laugh when I felt like crying and showed me that together we can face almost anything.

A Child of One's Own:
Some Thoughts on Birth and Adoption

Ellen Sarasohn Glazer

Several years ago, I was talking to a young boy about his family. When I asked him about siblings, he replied, "I have an older brother, Steven. We adopted him." In subsequent years, as my husband and I struggled to start a family of our own, I often thought about the boy's comment. I fantasized that I, too, would adopt a child and later become pregnant. I did not subscribe to the popular myth that adoption promoted fertility, but felt that at some point after we adopted, some medical or magical intervention would cause me to conceive. I imagined that this would lead to the worst of circumstances: one child who was an outsider in our family and another who was truly "our own." I expected that we would later regard the decision to adopt as a mistake.

I now have two daughters. Our older child, Elizabeth, came to us by adoption. Our younger child, Mollie, was born to us nearly three years later. I am now in the very "predicament" that I once feared. When I think back about the little boy and about my reaction to his comment, I cannot help but smile. I realize now that I understood so little at that time about attachments, about families, about the relationships that exist between parents and their children.

Elizabeth and Mollie are my children. I am well aware that they entered my life and our family in different ways. When they are old enough to know about these differences, they will certainly have feelings about them. However, what I did not know before I became their mother was that these differences would play a very small role in my perception of them and, at least at this point, in our ongoing experiences together. Moreover, I had no idea that the differences that do exist would add a valued dimension to our relationships.

When I have a quiet moment, and they are becoming increasingly scarce, I love to replay each of my daughter's arrivals. I try to re-run them in slow motion, giving myself a chance to enjoy moments which, at the time, went whizzing by. The deliveries, different in some ways, were each joyful experiences.

Elizabeth's arrival was announced by telephone. Don and I were sitting around one Sunday, planning our latest fertility strategy, when the phone rang. Don answered it and said, "Really, no shit!" Then he turned to me and said, "We have a daughter." I was startled. I thought for a moment about saying no and then suddenly found that I was ecstatic. In a frenzy I spent the next twenty-four hours making scattered attempts to prepare for our daughter's arrival. I stayed up all night and when she was finally delivered to us, I was too exhausted and too excited to look at her. I only remember a tiny bundle in yellow flowered bunting.

With Mollie, I stayed up all night, waiting for labor to begin. Having carried her for nine months, I had "known" that she was coming. However, my years of infertility had made it difficult for me to believe that she was ever really on her way. Even that night, as I paced the house in the same kind of scattered state that I was in awaiting Elizabeth, I did not have a clear sense that a baby would be born to us within twenty-four hours. When she was finally delivered, after ten hours of hard labor, I was too exhausted and too excited to look at her. Mollie and I really met several hours later. I went into the nursery and realized that I had no idea which baby was Mollie. As with Elizabeth, others had to tell me which child was mine. Each time, once told, the attachment began.

The attachment, whether to a biological or an adopted child, feels the same; the pride feels different. I have been aware, since Mollie arrived, that I take a more private delight in her than I do in Elizabeth. With Elizabeth, I burst with pride. It is public. It is unlimited. It is never self-conscious. I don't hesitate to tell anyone that I think she is beautiful, that I suspect she is "gifted," that I see her as the wittiest, most talented of children.

With Mollie, I "kvell" (a Yiddish expression meaning bursting with pride) silently. I see her as cute. I find her sweet, but I do not proclaim these thoughts publicly. Yesterday, I was changing her diaper with a friend and caught myself as I was about to say, "Oh, Mollie, you're so cute." Instead, I turned sheepishly to my friend and said, "I think that she is beginning to get cute."

The difference, as I see it, has to do with taking and giving credit. When I delight in Elizabeth, I never feel that I am bragging. I may know that I am, in part, responsible for who and what she is, but I don't feel it. When I admire her, it never feels as if I am admiring a part of myself. My public delight comes not only out of a sense of license, but also out of a feeling of commitment to her biological relatives. It is my effort, however futile, to include them, since they, too, would burst with pride if they could only know her. When I delight in Mollie it is very personal. I look at her fingers, her toes, and cannot quite believe that they developed inside me. I am guarded about taking credit because I am staggered and humbled.

From day to day, I do not think of my daughters as different. When I am battling with Elizabeth to get her dressed in the morning or in for a nap, I do not think of her adoption. She is mine, for better or for worse. When I am feeding Mollie, I do not think of her as my first-born. She is my younger child and will always remain so.

However, on occasions, particularly birthdays, there are differences—differences that I note and respect rather than regard as an intrusion. Mollie has not yet celebrated her first birthday. When she does, I expect it will be a happy occasion, one that will commemorate her arrival as well as celebrate her development at one year. I do not anticipate that it will be a very complicated occasion. Elizabeth's first birthday was a time of celebration but it was also a bittersweet occasion. As it approached I realized that the day she was born, March 24th, had little meaning for me; the day that I felt like celebrating was April 8th, the day that she came to our home. Moreover, I knew that on March 24th, there would be other people commemorating the day and that, for them, it would be a day without celebration. However, since her birthday is for her and not for them or for us, March 24th was, and has remained, the day upon which we rejoice.

Elizabeth's second and third birthdays have felt less complicated. April 8th has faded into the background, as have some of my concerns about her "other parents." March 24th is her day and I do all that I can to make it a special time for her. Nonetheless, the days between March 24th and April 8th remain a solemn time for me, an annual fifteen-day period in which I am very much aware that I was absent for my daughter's birth and early days. (Now these days take on additional meaning since they commemorate a time in which Mollie, too, was part of my life, but not yet known to me. Conceived on March 23rd, she announced her intentions by thermometer on April 8th).

Religious occasions, like birthdays, are a time in which I think about the differences in my daughters' origins. Mollie was born a Jew, will be raised as one, and will, I hope, find that her religion has something to offer. It is her birthright; there were no choices to be made. Elizabeth was born a Christian and was converted to Judaism when she was little over a month old. She had no say in the matter. We, as her parents, made a decision to take away one very rich heritage and to offer her another. Having made that decision, I feel it is my responsibility, as well as my pleasure, to offer her something in return. For Elizabeth, I hope that her religion will be special, that she will find it an enriching and satisfying part of her life. It is she to whom I sing in Hebrew, hoping that she will soon learn the words and the melodies.

When I was pregnant, I was very much aware that I was absent at Elizabeth's birth. I asked myself if I was sorry she wasn't my biological child, too. For her, and her future feelings, I wish that I could remove the fact of her adoption. For her other parents, excluded and undoubtedly in pain, I wish that they had not had to surrender their child. However, for myself, I do not wish that I had conceived, carried, and delivered her. What I missed prenatally and in those first fourteen days seems insignificant compared to the very special way in which she entered our family. Moreover, her delivery, so different from Mollie's and yet so similar, has added a special texture to the fabric of our lives.

The Adoption
Fran Castan

I remember the quiet room, the dark
green chair where we sat afternoons,
the sun—no matter how tightly shuttered out—
coming in and curving across us
as if we were not separate, but a single body
joined in a ceremony of light.
My legs beneath you, my arms around you,
my breast under the glass bottle with rubber nipple,
I talked to you and sang to you.
No one interrupted us.
The dog sat quietly in the corner.
If I could have given birth to you,
I would have. I would have taken you
inside me, held you
and given birth to you again.
All the hours we spent in that room. Then,
one day, with your eyes focused on mine, you
reached up and stroked my cheek. Your touch
was that of the inchworm on its aerial thread
just resting on my skin, a larval curve
alighting and lifting off, a lightness
practicing for the time it will have wings.
I like to think wherever you go, you will
keep some memory of sunlight in the room
where I first loved you, and you first loved.

14
Childfree Living

W HILE they are undergoing infertility diagnosis and treatment, most couples feel painfully childless. They are acutely aware that something is missing from their lives. They feel isolated and alone. Somewhere along the way, however, most of these couples decide that there are other avenues to parenthood, and they make decisions to adopt or attempt donor insemination, or perhaps even surrogate mothering. Yet there are some couples who identify a second choice that does not involve parenthood: they elect to live "childfree."

Childfree living is the term that is generally used to designate those couples who are infertile but have decided not to adopt. The term *childfree* is somewhat misleading since these couples are not necessarily free of children. In fact, children may even play a large part in their lives. What they feel free of is infertility. Childfree couples have chosen to put their infertility behind them and move on in their lives. Given the options available to them, they have decided that what is best for them is to live their lives without becoming parents.

The decision to be childfree does not often come easily to couples who have actively pursued infertility diagnosis and treatment. They must not only grieve the loss of their potential children, but they must also mourn the loss of the opportunity to parent together and to expand their family unit. They must accept that they will never have many of the experiences about which they had talked and fantasized.

It is sometimes difficult to understand why a couple, who very much wanted to be parents, would choose childfree living rather than adoption, or another parenting alternative. There are many reasons, though, why couples choose to be childfree. Sometimes reports of long waiting lists at adoption agencies scare them. They can't imagine waiting that long, or they feel that their efforts to adopt, like their efforts to conceive, will end in disappointment. Many of these couples do not have the financial means for a private or identified adoption and, unfortunately, their choice is sometimes made by default. Other couples decide not to adopt because of personal concerns about their ability or desire to parent an adopted child. These decisions to remain childfree are also made more by default than by a desire to be childfree.

Other couples actively decide to remain childfree. They see many positive reasons for not becoming parents, and believe that their family can be complete without children. Sometimes they are couples who have been together for a long time and have a history of being a family unit. They may have met and married later in life and for them, also, being a couple means being a family. Other couples who actively decide to remain childfree may have been married at a very young age and waited several years before attempting pregnancy. After many years of infertility, they are used to life without children. Despite the pain of infertility, they have settled into a comfortable life style and feel accepting of the childfree option.

The decision not to become parents can be difficult, especially if there is disagreement within the couple. One member may have a strong aversion to adoption while the other is interested in this option. Sometimes the spouse who wants to be childfree has had biological children by an earlier marriage, and feels no need to have any additional children, especially adopted ones. For these couples who have different desires, the process of identifying a second choice is particularly challenging and often painful.

When couples are unable to resolve their differences, and they remain childfree because one member is unwilling to adopt, a strain is inevitably put on their marriage. Resentment builds and tension mounts. The marriage itself may be at risk. It is important for all couples—but especially couples who have differences—to talk frequently and openly about their feelings. It is essential that they listen carefully to what their partner says, while trying not to feel threatened.

Those couples who are actively able to make a decision to be childfree usually express a great sense of relief. They report feeling increasingly comfortable around pregnant women and mothers with young children. They find that without doctor's appointments and treatment regimens, they have more time and energy to pursue other interests and move on with their lives. They are able to celebrate some of the rewards of life without children. Many also report finding satisfying ways of being with other people's children—nieces and nephews, children of friends, or children in need.

Couples who elect to be childfree are sometimes surprised to discover that they still have a good deal in common with couples who have children. Once parents have passed that period of time in which they are intensely involved in raising young children, they are free to again pursue more adult activities. Childfree couples often pursue friendships with couples who have older children, those no longer absorbed with maternity clothes or diapers.

Paradoxically, there is one group from whom those who choose childfree living may feel isolated: their infertile friends. Having neither achieved a successful pregnancy, nor chosen adoption, they are different from most of their infertile companions. Sometimes friends who have chosen to adopt may feel in a subtle way that their child is being rejected by the "childfree couple," and, as a result, both couples may distance themselves. Adoptive and prospective adoptive parents don't always realize that childfree couples are not rejecting their particular child—it is the alternative for themselves that they have rejected.

We have found that couples move from being childless to childfree in different ways. For some, the decision comes easily; for others it is made only after a long, hard struggle, and, unfortunately for still others, it is made by default. But the decision to remain childfree—though potentially a positive one, can feel unbearable if it is not made after careful thinking and soul-searching, and extensive communication between husband and wife.

Once the decision is made, however, the pain is not gone. The couple must grieve for the child whom they have not borne and who will not come to be. That dream child, though not real in flesh and blood, was a part of their longings for many years. He or she was a constant presence in their lives and they must mourn the loss. Although grieving can take time, we feel strongly that when couples give in to their feelings rather than fight them, the pain can be over. What remains is a feeling of sadness that usually stays in the background. Sometimes, particular events or thoughts can trigger it, but the emotion is more fleeting than in the past. And it is far more bearable.

In working with couples exploring childfree living, we encourage approaching the decision actively, carefully considering what it will mean for them now and in the future. We help them explore what parenthood means to them, and the extent to which a biological connection to their child is necessary. We try to help them understand whether not choosing adoption (or surrogate motherhood or donor insemination) means they have rejected non-biological parenting, or whether they are simply frightened of the process. We emphasize that those who decide to live childfree should be couples who truly regard it as a second choice.

We encourage those couples who decide to be childfree to consider how they can best make the transition from being childless to childfree. Sometimes we suggest that they make a tentative decision for a designated period of time—perhaps six months or a year. During that time they should share their thoughts and feelings with each other. And then, if the decision "feels" right, they can finalize it. We caution them about continuing to secretly hope for a pregnancy; it can only interfere with, and prolong, resolution. In fact, we encourage couples to use birth control, once they have made the decision to be childfree. Often the man elects to have a vasectomy, or the woman to have her tubes tied.

In "A Couple Family," Martha Maxfield shares with the reader the process by which she and her husband decided to remain childfree. Though she still feels sad from time to time, she is very clear that the decision was the right one for them.

A Couple Family:
The Decision to Remain Childfree

Martha Maxfield

It has been nine years since we decided to stay a childfree family. There have been major changes in our expectations for the future. During our seven years of trying to conceive, we had occasionally discussed the possibility of not having children. It was part of coping with month after month of nonpregnancy.

Like most women raised in the fifties and sixties, I had the usual expectations of marriage, children, a home of our own, a part-time job. My career in nursing fulfilled the future part-time job; I met and married a wonderful man; and we decided to wait two years before starting our family. On our second anniversary, we stopped using birth control and started discussing names for our soon-to-be child. Five and a half years later, after on-and-off infertility testing, we decided to give it one last attempt, and devote one full year to concentrated testing. By the end of that year, I was emotionally spent, working closely with co-workers who were pregnant, and still not pregnant myself. I was sick of being in limbo and of answering "we're trying," when asked about starting our family. After all the years, that statement was wearing thin.

Our first contact with other infertile couples was through an ad for a six-week workshop sponsored by a community center. It was a great help to be able to talk with others going through the same tests, and feeling the same stresses that we were. We were finally able to talk with others about our anger and frustrations, and they understood. It was during this time that we reached our decision to remain childfree.

We did not reach that decision overnight. Nor was it easy. Nor did it immediately solve all our emotional stress. It had begun to evolve over the years of non-pregnancy. I've occasionally been accused of not having wanted a child very much in the first place. *Not true!* I wanted Bill's child so badly I ached for it. I wanted to go through a pregnancy with a child conceived and born of our love. Making the decision to give up trying was not easy.

There are many factors involved. Emotionally, I couldn't take much more testing and treatment that might or might not work. Our age was also becoming a concern to us. I think most every couple has a target age for becoming parents beyond which they prefer not to go. My first one was twenty-five, and I was already several years beyond that. I did not want to be an "older parent." We wanted to be able to visualize a time of financial freedom—when we would be young enough to enjoy it. We had heavy financial responsibilities for the first ten to twelve years of our marriage, and we wanted to be able to see an end to that.

When we finally sat down to seriously consider remaining childfree, we made a list: why we wanted children; why we might wish to remain childfree. The childfree side outweighed the other. The most important reason then and now is that our relationship does not need a child to complete it or fulfill it; we are very happy as a couple. We talked about it over and over for several days. We kept asking ourselves if we were making the right decision.

We never considered adoption. There is no real reason why; it is just something neither of us wished to pursue. For myself, the child I wanted was Bill's child—to go through a pregnancy and birth together. This is Bill's second marriage; he has two children from his first. He had the financial support of them, but few of the pleasures of fatherhood. My feelings for his children are the same I have for my neices and nephews. I love them dearly, but they are not our biological children—the product of our love. Both of us felt the pain of not being able to have a child of our own.

The decision to remain childfree ushered in the worst period of my life. My unborn child, who I had named and who was the object of my fantasies, was dead. My whole future had been planned around motherhood and now it was a blank. I was grieving for my loss, but no one could understand. Unfortunately, it was two to three months before the local RESOLVE chapter was started and a support group was available to us.

We had to go through the grieving process, which included feeling angry, and lashing out at others, until we finally came to truly accept our decision. For years, our lives had revolved around temperature charts, doctor's visits, and timing; now there was nothing but us. Like any major loss, it took several months to heal. And, as difficult as it was, I never considered reversing the decision and continuing the infertility testing. Things did get easier when we got into a support group with others who could understand our loss. For even though the people in our group did not elect to remain childfree, they were very supportive and understanding.

Several months after our decision, we made plans to finalize it. Since I had had difficult menstrual periods, I decided to undergo a hysterectomy. The surgeon discovered I had endometriosis, so we had an answer of sorts about why I couldn't get pregnant. I was not depressed after surgery; if anything, I was happy. Since we had never been given a diagnosis for our infertility, there was always the possibility I might conceive. After going through the pain of grieving, and finally healing, I did not want to find myself pregnant in my late thirties. The hysterectomy freed me of this possibility.

Many positive changes accompanied being childfree. One change is financial security. We have only ourselves to support. We don't have to plan for child care or clothing or college tuition. Being childfree has given me the freedom to step back and make career decisions. I work part-time as a nurse, part-time as a craftsperson, and do volunteer work. Another positive change is that we recovered our sexual spontaneity. Years of temperature charts and sex on demand had taken its toll on our sex life. It was wonderful to recapture that intimacy.

What hasn't changed is us. We started out as a couple and we remain a couple. Our relationship has only gotten better over the years. We present ourselves as a couple family. Just because we have no children, we're still a solid family.

My regrets are fleeting and infrequent. The feelings of loss for my unborn child are similar to the ones I have for my grandmother and other important people who have died. There are happenings—a song, a sunset, for example, that remind me of them, and I feel a pang that they are not here to share life with me. My infertility has had a big influence on my life and will always be with me, but it does not rule my life. I can go to baby showers and outings with children and enjoy myself very much. When things get noisy, as they inevitably do, I know that I can return to the quiet of my house.

I decided many years ago that I was not going to live my life with regrets and *if onlys*. Trying to undo the past would leave me no time to enjoy the present. I am busy, content, and feel very fulfilled. There are, however, many things I would like to do for which I just do not have time. Perhaps I will in the future.

Our marriage has weathered sixteen years, and everything we have gone through has made our relationship stronger. Being a childfree family is not for everyone, but it has been the right choice for us.

15
Parenting after Infertility

W HEN a child arrives, whether it be by birth or adoption, most infertile parents are filled with delight. Not only do they have a child to be with and care for, but they have also been freed from childlessness. Their isolation is gone and they pass their first few weeks and months as parents in a sleepless, blissful daze with infertility (almost) forgotten.

Before too long, however, infertility again rears its angry head. Unless a couple plans to have only one child, infertile parents soon recognize that while their lives may feel fuller, and certainly busier, their family is incomplete. Once again, they are reminded that they are different from fertile parents. They cannot afford to wait until they are ready to begin trying to conceive or to adopt a second child. They must risk having a second child "too soon" because they know, all too well, that they may have to wait too long. This need to consider a second child, before they are ready, may rob parents of the chance to fully delight in their first child.

While they are first undergoing infertility diagnosis and treatment, many couples engage in a bargaining process, which goes something like this, "If I am ever able to have a child, I will do my very best. I promise never to complain. I won't resent the child. On my honor, I promise never, ever, to raise my voice." And on it goes.

Now these earnest bargainers have become parents. They may have a toddler who pulls all the cans off the shelf in the supermarket, or a three-year-old who has a tantrum because she wants to make her own lunch. Promises have been made that are hard to keep. Infertile parents sometimes feel as if they have made a deal with the devil.

Infertile couples who promised to be superparents, look around them at the shortcomings of other parents and continue to feel different. They resent having to demand so much of themselves, and fear the consequences, should they abandon their vigilance. This feeling is heightened for adoptive parents who, as part of the adoption process, had to prove themselves highly worthy of being parents.

As all parents know, their children begin to separate from them at an early age. Each developmental milestone—crawling, walking, speaking—is evidence of the child's growing independence, of her increased ability to function alone in the world. By a very early age, often even before toilet training, children declare "I can do it by myself." Parents usually delight in their children's accomplishments, and take pride in their mastery. For infertile parents, a child's movement toward separation is often a more ambivalent experience. Because they do not live with the assumption that they can have more children, they may be more vulnerable to feelings of loss as they watch their child grow. Fertile parents often acknowledge holding on to their youngest child, keeping him a baby longer because he will be their last. Infertile parents report having those feelings with each of their children.

Fertile parents have a reference point of childfree living; couples who knew long-term infertility remember only childlessness. This imprint of childlessness not only affects parents' feelings about their children's growth and development, but it also has an impact on their behavior. Frequently, they report having difficulties disciplining their children. Though they recognize, in the abstract, that limits are essential, they may find it hard to set them with a child who is so special.

The imprint of childlessness compromises parents' ability to be separated from their children, particularly when they are young. Some have trouble leaving them with babysitters or in day care, finding it difficult to return to jobs that they want or need to resume. Others find it hard to be together as a couple, away from their child, for it is painfully reminiscent of their childless state. Sometimes infertile parents are overly protective, fearing that without their constant vigilance something terrible will happen. They may recognize that being too concerned or watchful can interfere with their child's growth and development, but the threat of loss remains real to them. They know that children can never be replaced.

Infertile parents' struggles are further complicated by the fact that they are often older parents. Some face menopause or the onset of medical problems when they have very young children. Many face their own parents' illnesses or deaths at this time. These changes bring real losses at a time when they are already struggling with fears and feelings of loss in relation to their children. A long awaited child may become even more special—for better or for worse—at a time when a woman recognizes the onset of menopause or a man loses his father.

Finally, many infertile parents live with a sense that their families are incomplete. Even in the presence of young children, they continue to suffer the loss of a child never born or of an adoption that fell through. Also, those that bear children report feeling an "addiction to fertility." Even when their families are sensibly complete, they are tempted to have more children to see if they can still get pregnant. Some actually enlarge their families, even when their better judgment advises them not to.

Adoptive parents, as we mentioned earlier, have additional role handicaps. They are likely to feel especially vulnerable to loss, fearing that someday their child and his or her birthparent will claim each other. Or they fear that others—or they themselves—will be critical of their ability to parent. Adoptive parents are often startled to find that while their child fulfills much of their need to be a parent, they still feel biologically defective and left out. Often it seems that biological parents belong to a special club—one that continually discusses labor, delivery, and breast feeding—and to which they are forever denied membership.

In working with parents after infertility, we try to help them see that they have not, in fact, made a deal with devil. Attempts to be superparents simply prolong the pain of infertility, emphasizing differences, rather than commonalities. Instead, infertile parents need permission to complain, to feel disappointed, or to be angry, and most important, to acknowledge that parenthood is not always the blissful state they imagined it would be.

We try, also, to help parents develop a childfree reference point. With encouragement, they can begin to enjoy an evening out or feel comfortable returning to work or to other adult activities. Memories of childlessness remain powerful, but infertile parents do find that separations are necessary for their child's growth and development, as well as for their own.

Finally, we try to help infertile parents appreciate some of the advantages of their experience. Because they can never take their children for granted, they live with a sense of wonder. For them, the arrival of a child in their lives, whether it be by birth or adoption, is truly a miracle. And the imprint of childlessness, while sometimes a burden, can also be a blessing. At the worst moments—when their children are their most difficult selves and parents are suffering from terminal frustration, it is truly a gift to be able to call childlessness to mind. A two-year-old's worst tantrum is but a mild annoyance to someone who remembers being on an emotional roller coaster from month to month.

In the pages that follow, four women look back on their infertility and consider the legacy that it has left behind. In "Overprotectiveness: A Result of Infertility?" Peggy Cramer chronicles the struggles she experiences being the mother of an only child born after years of infertility. Amy Shoenbrun confesses to some of the frustrating realities of parenting in "And Be Ye Eternally Grateful." Dorothy Allen, in "The Hardest Job I've Ever Done," describes the ambivalence, as well as joy, that she feels as a mother. Finally, Carol Schraft, mother of three older children—one adopted and two biological—reflects back on her sixteen years of parenting after infertility. She offers wisdom and hindsight about the importance of accepting and loving our children, with all their strengths and weaknesses, no matter how they came to us.

Overprotectiveness:
A Result of Infertility?

Peggy Cramer

Me, overprotective of our only child? You can bet on it—or at least in my every thought, but hopefully not in my behavior. It's not easy living with the conflict of feelings and behavior, but I do, for the well being of both of us.

After six years of infertility we celebrated our first pregnancy. Protective feelings emerged in me from the day the test was positive. Should I continue to work? Should I continue to play tennis and racquetball? Though I agonized at length about these questions, for me the answer was *yes*. In an effort to quell the rising tide of anxiety and apprehension, I tried to appear normal to the outside world. Maybe I overdid it a little by playing racquetball when I was eight months along!

If the protective urge was present during my pregnancy, it was quadrupled after an emergency Caesarian saved both our lives. While still in the hospital I can remember thinking, "how can I ever send J.J. to kindergarten?" I also understood for the first time the reasons why parents have thrown themselves in front of moving vehicles to save their children. I thus became aware of my strong overprotective urges, and resolved to temper them with what I believed was normal behavior.

When our son was one and a half, I decided to do substitute teaching. I found good day care for J.J.—a woman who was willing to take him on a substitute's haphazard schedule. I rationalized my feelings by saying that since he was an only child, the exposure to other children was good for him. Fortunately, he parted from me easily, though my feelings were mixed about leaving him.

Later, J.J. was ready for school. In our school system, all kindergarten children are bused to school. I could have driven him, but decided he should do what all the others do—the normal once again. We waited together at the bus stop and I took pictures of him in his new school clothes. When he and the bus were out of sight, I cried. But I felt I was doing the right thing for both of us.

When he was in second grade he was eligible to ride his bike to school. J.J., of course, wanted to, while I was torn by my fears of possible danger. We compromised. First, we walked the route he would ride, choosing the safest paths, and pointing out the most dangerous intersections. The first time he took off on his bike I watched from the window until he was out of sight. Though I had the urge to get in the car and follow him, I prayed instead for his safety.

These are just a few examples of the times in our twelve years together that I was able to make the right decision for J.J., contrary to an inward pull to hold onto him a little longer, a little closer, a little tighter. The hardest times of all are when he is sick. Even with good medical care, the emotional strain of simply waiting it out is agonizing. I am constantly fearful that he will be seized from me. I tell myself that all parents feel this way when their children are sick, but I'm not sure I believe it.

Through the years, my strong overprotective urges have been tempered by wanting to do what I felt was really best for my son. And I guess it has been best for me, too. I have learned to let go slowly, in little tiny steps. First, leaving him with a baby sitter, then sending him off to school, later allowing him to ride a bike, then letting him stay overnight at a friend's house, and finally sending him to overnight camp for a week. Each step taken has proven to me that I can manage his growing independence with maturity, and with somewhat less difficulty.

All these earlier challenges to my ability to let go could be anticipated. They are part of normal growth and development—steps that every parent must go through, although perhaps with less difficulty than I did. Recently, however, I was faced with a challenge for which I was unprepared.

At twelve, J.J. is a talented and ambitious tennis player. He loves the game and has hopes of being a professional tennis player. In order to do this he needs to have frequent opportunities to play with boys of equal or better skill, and he needs constant instruction. A boarding school would offer him this opportunity.

J.J. wants very much to go away to school, and I have sensibly but reluctantly said *yes*. I made this decision because I realized that his reasons were sound, and that it would not be in his best interest to hold him back. Still, it was, and remains, a painful process for me. I feel I will be missing out on much of his adolescence, losing years we could have shared together. I realize now that my six years of infertility do not entitle me to special parental rights. Like mothers before me, and those that will follow, I must let go before I am ready.

And Be Ye Eternally Grateful

Amy Shoenbrun

When my daughters were ages two-and-a-half years and two-and-a-half weeks, we spent one memorable morning in the dentist's chair together. I had unwittingly scheduled my older daughter Emily's first dental exam to occur just after her sister Sally's arrival. Worse still, I had made the appointment for 8:00 A.M., having no idea that it is one thing to get an adult to an early appointment, and entirely another to manage it with a toddler and an infant.

Emily, Sally, and I made a crash landing at Dr. S's office. Since Emily is a very independent little girl, and since she was particularly proud—or so it seemed—to be a big sister, I had not anticipated a problem with the exam. Hence, it was a surprise for me when Emily let out a blood curdling shriek and tried to run out the front door.

I won't go into the details of how we arranged seating, but it turned out that the only way Dr. S could get Emily into the chair was to have her on my lap, which of course meant having her next to Sally, who was always on my lap those days. Nor will I go into the record number of diaper changes that Sally needed during that eternal forty-five minutes. I will mention, however, that Emily vomited all over Sally's Snugli and Dr. S's shoes.

My fertile friends would surely regard this episode as a nightmare. For me, after years of infertility, it was a mild inconvenience, in some ways even enjoyable. I remember looking up at Dr. S's puzzled face and thinking, "He should only know what I went through to become a mother. He should only know what these children mean to me."

Several years have passed and my daughters are now nearly seven and five. I look back on this incident and on the several hundred less dramatic ones that have occurred throughout these years. I am aware of the impact that my infertility has had on my experiences as a mother. On the one hand, it has given me valuable perspective, one that enables me to accept—even embrace—dreadful moments like when Emily's vomit landed on Dr. S's shoes. At the same time, however, infertility has also left me with certain burdens that make motherhood more complicated and more difficult.

"Be ye eternally grateful," my infertility tells me. "Remember how much you wanted these children. Cherish them. Do not take them for granted. Remember never to complain," and on it goes. My infertility limits my ability to express frustration and disappointment and, at times, it has kept me locked into a system of magical thinking. Sometimes, I feel that I've signed an imaginary contract that commits me to gratitude. Should I ease up on my side of the bargain, I face that most feared of punishments: the loss of my children.

I did ease up once recently, and the experience was an unsettling but necessary one. The girls and I were in the Orlando airport returning home from a week at Disneyworld. They were playing happily, but noisily, as we waited for our plane, now two hours late. As they hopped, skipped, jumped, danced about, vying for my attention, I found myself growing increasingly impatient with them. Worse yet, I was intolerant of my own intolerance. They were just being kids—good kids, in fact—and I was being an ungrateful mother. A man sitting nearby said, "Mom, I can tell you've had it."

I responded, "I sure have. I can't wait until they go back to school." The words slipped out. When I heard them I felt jolted. I had broken the contract—I had gone public with my ingratitude. There was a moment of fear, but it was followed by a sense of relief.

Here, at the seven year mark, I think I am beginning to make a truce with my infertility. I am starting to acknowledge, however hesitantly, that motherhood is not exactly the promised land. I adore my daughters, and they are a source of great joy and satisfaction. Still, being their mother can be frustrating and exhausting. It is a job well worth doing, but not always a dream come true.

The Hardest Job I've Ever Done

Dorothy Allen

During the long period of my infertility, I never once thought about being a mother. What I thought about constantly was having a baby. Somehow this baby never grew up; in fact, she never did a lot of things—like whine or talk back or refuse to listen to me. The point is that I had no idea what the job of parenthood really entailed. I had no idea what the emotional commitment was all about. I assumed the task would be easy. The only entrance exam required was fertility, and I believed if I could get beyond that I would have it made. After all, I reasoned, I was approaching thirty, had a few years of psychotherapy behind me, a decent marriage, a master's degree, a good job, and had done some traveling. In short, I felt ready to "relax" and enjoy the blissful experience of motherhood, which I believed consisted of the sweet smell of talcum and a happy gurgling baby. My children are now eleven and seven, and those smells and sounds are a distant memory.

Motherhood has been an ambivalent state for me during these eleven years. I have experienced moments of bliss—like when my daughter crept silently behind me the other day, planted a kiss on my cheek, and told me she loved me. And I have experienced moments of utter misery—like when she told me I was the meanest mommy in the whole world and she wanted me to get a divorce so she could live with daddy. Both my children have "strong" personalities, which is to say they are independent, stubborn, direct, articulate, bossy, self-confident, and curious. I love these attributes and I hate them. I loved that my son felt ready this past summer to go to overnight camp and I love it that he wants to go on the scary amusement park rides with me. But I hate it when he won't read directions to a new game because he's convinced he can figure it out by looking at the board, or when he tries to get me to change my mind after I've already said *no* four times.

There are only two facts, seemingly paradoxical, about which I am very certain. One is that if either one of my children died or was taken away from me, I would never get out of bed again. I know that I could not go on living. Surely, I would never smile any more. The second fact is that if I knew twelve years ago what I know today, I might have decided not to have children. Certainly the lists, pro and con, would be about equal in length.

When I was infertile it did not occur to me that I would have babies who would grow up into children, who would grow up into teenagers. And it did not occur to me that they might also develop—by virtue of heredity or upbringing, I have not yet decided which—some of my own most disliked traits. If I weren't so independent, stubborn, direct, articulate, bossy, self-confident, and curious, we would probably rarely clash. And some of the most painful realizations I have experienced as a mother, are the ways in which I am like my own parents. It is their negative characteristics, not the positive ones, that wave before my eyes like flags on a windy day.

In watching my children grow up, and in being an active participant in that process, I have discovered, to my dismay, that I am not the nice person I thought I was. Nor would I qualify in any way for the Mental Health of the Year Award. Among my unfortunate discoveries is a tenacity that I didn't know existed; I lack patience much of the time, I scream a lot, and at least a handful of times I have been mildly physically abusive. Emotionally, I have often felt out of control. When I remember my infertility experience I sometimes feel ashamed, believing it was a sign from God that I would be an unfit mother. When I can get some distance from my negative perceptions I sometimes play a game with my children. It goes like this: "Just before your next life, when you're up in heaven, tell God you want a mother with much more patience than the last one." Or, "Tell God you want a mother who will let you stay up as late as you want at night."

My image of myself as a mother is not all terrible. I do some things quite well. For example, I make up clever bedtime stories that have just the right moral for that day's mishap. I'm good at comforting my children when their feelings have been hurt. I'm open about my own experiences and feelings, can easily talk to them about love and sex, and am physically affectionate. When I'm feeling good about my interactions with my children, it all seems worth it. At those times the game goes like this, "When you're up in heaven, just before your next life, tell God you want a mommy who is as great a story teller as this one." Or, "Tell God you want a mommy who bakes chocolate cake as good as I do."

Actually, motherhood is teaching me a lesson similar to the one that infertility taught me. It's about control. I can't always be what I want, and I can't always have what I want. Although I don't like some things about myself as a mother, I am learning to accept myself, while at the same time, trying to do better. My children are not always who I would want them to be, but I am doing my best to accept them for who they are. Loving them, of course, was never an issue.

Mothering is the most difficult job I have ever done—more difficult than writing my doctoral thesis; more difficult even than learning statistics. I have encountered the best and the worst of myself. At times I have regretted the job immensely and experienced great sadness, like last week when my son in his anger said, "In my next life I hope I have a mom who understands kids." At other times, the job is delightful and my children make me laugh, like tonight, when my daughter, glumfaced, looked up from her broccoli and said, "In my next life, I'm going to ask God for a mother who won't make me eat my vegetables." Motherhood has indeed been an ambivalent state.

Looking Back

Carol Schraft

The story of our infertility is so much like the others. There were several years of tests, drugs, temperature charts, surgery, more tests, new drugs. It was a long, anxious, often embarrassing, unhappy time. Yet, as I write about those events now, nearly twenty years later, it is hard to recapture them. I can see the temperature charts roughly drawn with an odd collection of ball point pens; I can describe the hospital room that was, as requested, on the surgical rather than the Ob-Gyn floor. I can tell you about the hours passed with outdated magazines in the waiting room of Yale-New Haven Hospital Infertility Clinic. But the experience itself is complete, finished, an historical event devoid of life, safe in the archives.

The story of our children is, as I am frequently told, so much like the stories of others like my husband and me. That is, we adopted a child; within a few weeks I became pregnant; and, after the birth of that child, unexpectedly pregnant again. So, we went quickly from the years of longing for a single peaceful child to a noisy, somewhat chaotic household strewn with cartons of Pampers and what seemed like the complete line of Fisher-Price toys.

For fifteen years, the Pavlovian response to the story of how our family came to be has been, "That's what happens all the time," followed by an account of a second cousin or a friend of a friend who adopted a child and immediately found themselves pregnant. While I have come to believe this bit of conventional wisdom, much the way I believe that a stitch in time saves nine, I have never actually met, or even talked on the phone, to a person who adopted a child and soon after gave birth to another. I do think this last bit unusual, given the fact that I was first a social worker and am now an elementary school principal, and in nearly a quarter century of working life, have met what by now must number thousands of parents.

I doubt that my experience of pregnancy after adoption happens with the frequency imagined. I would guess that it occurs with the same frequency as does pregnancy after many years of infertility. I suspect, however, that the myth is popular as a way, albeit well-intentioned, of trivializing infertility, or making it a psychological problem that clears up as soon as you just calm down and relax. This is a point of view that helps no one, least of all a woman unable to conceive. The arena of infertility is filled with beliefs and "mother wit" that cloud an already miserable condition. In fostering the point of view that the most common occurrence after adoption is conception, one fosters the belief that infertility is primarily in the head.

Other common beliefs about infertility have to do with genetics. In trying to overcome infertility, one is making a statement about the importance of genetics; in choosing adoption, one is making a statement about the importance of upbringing. Either way, we, as potential parents, are central to an unfolding drama as either biological or social engineer. With that disclaimer, impressions of my own experience follow.

I remember the period of my own infertility, so long ago, in an intellectual way, but empty of feeling. Often I have talked about it, in what I hope has been a helpful manner, to others struggling with childlessness. As with all struggles, however, I believe that it is transitory. No matter how many years, how many pills and injections and surgical procedures, how many cycles counted day by unending day, infertility must eventually be resolved either by bearing a biological child, adopting, or remaining childfree. My own resolution, though, was not nearly as important to me as the realization preceding it that my life could not continue forever in an obsessive concern with reproduction. I finally had to let go, move on, and allow infertility to take its rightful place in my memory, no longer draining energy from day to day life.

Our particular resolution to infertility was adoption—an event recalled from the heart. I can remember no happier time than when we adopted our daughter, our first child. Although I have never been a religious person, a friend recently told me that I described her as "a gift from heaven." That sense of complete love and exhilaration, of overflowing with joy is what, I believe, the literature has come to call bonding. To me it felt like a spiritual transformation. I am well aware, though, that the counterweight to our happiness was probably sadness beyond any that I can even imagine for our daughter's biological mother.

Shortly after adoption I ovulated. Whether my joy in being a mother had some impact on my hypothalamus, or whether it was some fluke of nature, does not matter. What is important in the history of our family is that one son and then another was born. During all those years of waiting, fantasies about what it would be like to have children had ample time and a fertile imagination in which to grow. Interestingly, my imaginary children never grew to be more than two or, at the most, three years old. They were very attractive, cheerful, well-dressed, well-behaved. They never cried, fought with one another, had tantrums or fevers of 105 at 3:20 in the morning. These longed-for fantasy children were not, in fact, real children at all, but rather loving and complimentary extensions of my husband and me.

Our real children—all three—though similar in cosmetic ways, have turned into people with unalterable traits that "just are." One is outgoing, one is shy, and the other cautious. Two are excellent students, another dislikes school. One is almost compulsively neat, the others slovenly. One is a superb athlete, another average, and the other can barely catch a ball. Two have gourmet palates, another is strictly burgers and fries. One loves basketball, another Shakespeare, and the third loves tennis. Learning to live with these traits that "just are" is, in my experience, at the heart of parenthood. Sometimes it has been delightful, sometimes it has been maddening, sometimes it has caused nights without sleep. But the essence of parenting has been raising people different from me and learning to live with the inability to control or alter the way they "just are."

Having been a parent for nearly sixteen years, I now see how little I understood about it when this all began. Yes, the wish to leave one's mark on the world is very powerful. But it is also easy to forget that as parents, our darkest sides get recreated right along with our best, or that an adopted child comes from a place we probably will never know. Even when our children are biologically ours, they are still strangers when they arrive.

In the end, it doesn't matter so much how the children got there. It doesn't really matter whether you take them for swimming lessons or take them to the playground; whether you let them watch cartoons or restrict them to "Mr. Rogers." What does matter is your ability to love and accept them, whatever they look like, however they are.

About the Authors

ELLEN SARASOHN GLAZER is a clinical social worker in private practice working with individuals and couples experiencing infertility and/or exploring adoption. She is also on the staff of the psychiatry department at the Mt. Auburn Hospital in Cambridge, Massachusetts, and has been involved for many years with RESOLVE, Inc., as a past board member and current active member. She is a group leader for the Bay State Chapter of RESOLVE, Inc., facilitating both pre-adoption and infertility support groups. In addition, she is the author of several articles on parenting. Ms. Glazer lives in Newton, Massachusetts, with her two daughters, Elizabeth and Mollie.

SUSAN LEWIS COOPER is a psychologist and Codirector of Focus Counseling and Consultation, Inc., Cambridge, Massachusetts, where she works with individuals, couples, and families. After completing her doctoral dissertation at Boston University in 1979 on the emotional effects of infertility, she became actively involved with RESOLVE, Inc., and has served as a national board member for the past five years. She is a support group leader for RESOLVE of the Bay State, and has worked with individuals and couples experiencing both primary and secondary infertility. She is the coauthor of *Preparing, Designing, and Leading Workshops: A Humanistic Approach* (Van Nostrand Reinhold, 1980). Dr. Cooper lives in Brookline, Massachusetts, with her husband, Marc, and two children, Seth and Amanda.